Exercise Physiology

This book is one of a series on physical education edited by

Prof. John E. Kane

Principal, Loughborough College of Education

Other titles in this series include

The Mechanics of Human Movement by B. J. Hopper
Curriculum Development in Physical Education edited by John E. Kane

Other books by Vaughan Thomas

Science and Sport
Basketball: Techniques and Tactics

Exercise Physiology

Vaughan Thomas, Ph.D.

Crosby Lockwood Staples   London

Granada Publishing Limited
First published in Great Britain 1975 by
Crosby Lockwood Staples
Frogmore St Albans Hertfordshire AL2 2NF and
3 Upper James Street London W1R 4BP

ISBN 0 258 96901 6 (hardback)

Filmset in Photon Times 12 pt by
Richard Clay (The Chaucer Press), Ltd, Bungay, Suffolk
and printed in Great Britain by
Fletcher & Son Ltd, Norwich

Acknowledgements

This book would not have seen the light of day were it not for the enthusiasm and sagacity of the series editor, Dr John Kane; the foresight of Crosby Lockwood Staples in deciding to produce the series; the unfailing support and encouragement of my wife and children during my hours of blood-sweating incarceration; and the formulative influences of my own mentors, Professor Peter Davies of Surrey University, Dr Ernest Hamley of Loughborough University and Dr Henry Evans Robson of Loughborough College. I give them my thanks.

Also, the book could not have been written without the efforts of my parents in producing and rearing me – and I should like belatedly to express my affectionate appreciation to them by dedicating this work to Gwendoline and Harold Thomas.

The following illustrations are based on originals from other works, for which permission is gratefully acknowledged: 1.3, 1.4, 1:6, 1.7, 2.2, 2.3, 2.4, 2.5, 2.9, 2.11, 3.5, 4.1, 4.2, 4.3, 4.4, 4.5, 5.1, 5.2, 5.3, 5.5, 5.6, 5.7, 6.8, 6.12, 6.18, 6.20, 6.24, 6.26 – A. C. Guyton: *Function of the Human Body*. 3rd edition. W. B. Saunders Co., London, 1972.

2.1, 6.16, 6.17, 6.19 – A. B. McNaught and R. Callander: *Nurses' Illustrated Physiology*. E. & S. Livingstone, London, 1964.

2.13, 6.15 – Samson Wright: *Applied Physiology*. 12th edition, revised C. A. Keele and E. Neil. Oxford Medical Publications, London, 1971.

1.1 – W. D. McElroy: *Cell Physiology and Biochemistry*. 3rd edition. Foundations of Modern Biology series. Prentice-Hall, London, 1971.

Contents

Foreword

In the continuing development of a science of physical education and sport, the study of exercise physiology has for a long time represented the central hope for a disciplined link between derived knowledge of the body's functional adaptation and the practices forming the training curricula. Increasingly the implications of current knowledge for practices have been emphasised, but the relationship of knowledge to practice is essentially a changing one reflecting new researches and findings. Indeed the application of scientific knowledge and methods to athletic training is quite a recent development, as may be inferred from the following excerpt from the training routine of the Yale University crew in 1866:

> The crew rose each morning at six and then, in heavy flannels, ran from three to six miles on empty stomachs; in the forenoon they would row from four to six miles and do the same distance in the afternoon, and these rows were not easy paddles but hard, stiff trials and mostly on time. They ate underdone beef and mutton with the blood running from it, with a few potatoes or rice now and then, but no other vegetables, and drank weak tea in small quantities.

Since the taking of water was apt to put back the weight that had been lost through perspiration, the men were given only what they positively could not do without, and the agony of such a course when the men were rowing in the hot sun and perspiring freely can be imagined, and it was further increased by the prohibition of baths; some coaches would not permit their men to bathe for three weeks or more before a race.*

To many the identification of exercise physiology as a division of physiology dates from Professor A. V. Hill's presidential address to the Physiological Section of the British Association for the Advancement of Science, at its ninety-third convention in Southampton in 1925. Since then much new information has become available to give greater insights into the adaptation of the body during exercise, and this book by Dr Vaughan Thomas represents a synthesis and interpretation of current knowledge in this area. The book, which is the second in the Crosby Lockwood Staples Physical Education series, will appeal particularly to students of physical education and sports science, but its scope raises important issues of relevance to all those who, in one way or another, are interested in the limitations and integrative nature of human efficiency.

Dr Vaughan Thomas invests this work with a special combination of insights. Not only can he draw on his expertise as a physiologist, but he has also a very deep understanding of athletic sports by virtue of a wide-ranging and outstanding involvement as a practising athlete.

J. E. Kane

Loughborough College of Education

* As reported by Crowther and Ruhl in *Rowing and Track Athletics*, The Macmillan Company, 1905.

Introduction

This book is about the functioning of the human body in sports, games and recreative physical activities. It sets out to explain in simple terms what happens when we eat, drink, work and rest, and how to use the body to obtain the best performance of which it is capable. There have been many texts on exercise physiology – some of which are outstanding – written by physiologists. I am a sports ergonomist: sportsman first, scientist second. There is no physiology for its own sake within these pages though the fundamental concepts are treated briefly, because they directly affect the human as a sportsman.

The book will be of use to students of physical education, sports coaching and recreation provision. It covers the major part, if not all, of a physiology specialisation within a first degree course in physical education. In conjunction with a basic biochemistry text it would act as a suitable framework for a physiology option in a sports science degree course.

Chapter 1 is written to help those who lack a good school background in human biology. Some may prefer to read next the final chapter on adaptation, at least cursorily. They will then be able to see each chapter in a general framework. Since each chapter is devoted to one body system they may be taken in any order, though I believe the present order to be most helpful.

Over 300 references are made directly to research papers or standard reference works and in some cases students should refer to the primary source for fuller information. I acknowledge, moreover, my debt to the great body of knowledge won by exercise physiologists and hope to have assembled and integrated it in a form which can efficiently assist the understanding of exercise physiology.

To avoid repetition and unnecessarily lengthening the book (and increasing its price), the principle of cross referring is generally used. This should cause little inconvenience to the reader, and serves the additional purpose of integrating the various sections of the text.

Vaughan Thomas

Director of Physical Education,
Department of Physical Education,
Liverpool Polytechnic

Fundamental Physiology

When considering the functioning of the sportsman or sportswoman it is necessary first to understand the basis of all human functioning, that is, cellular function. The cells of the sportsman are in essence the same as the cells of anyone else, obeying the same laws, subject to the same effects. Subsequent chapters of the book are devoted to an analysis of what makes the sportsman *different*. This chapter looks at what he has in common – the nature of his cells – and is mainly concerned with those elements which affect sports function.

The cell

Human cells vary in size and form, but all are characterised by the presence of a *nucleus* surrounded by a *membrane* within the *cytoplasm*, the whole being encapsulated in another membrane. Also within the cytoplasm are smaller structures (mitochondria, ribosomes, lysosomes and the endoplasmic reticulum). A typical cell is illustrated in Fig. 1.1.

When a cell is placed in a suitably balanced nutrient, it is able to divide into two similar cells, a process called *mitosis*.

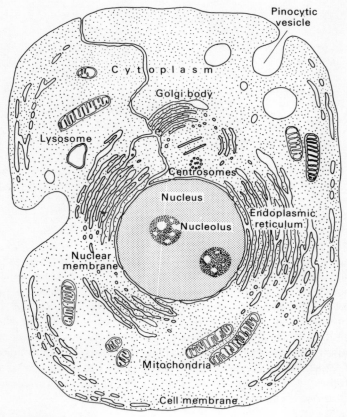

Fig. 1.1 A typical cell

Unless inhibited, mitosis occurs regularly at an interval between 10 and 30 hours.

Transport mechanisms

The cell membrane is the route through which all substances must pass when entering or leaving the cell. The membrane is selective, as also are the membranes of the intracellular structures, and therefore controls the passage of different substances at different times. The permeability of the membrane is not constant, being affected by many factors, including kind and concentration of ions, hormones, acidity and temperature.

The transport of a substance across a membrane takes place by several mechanisms, subject to different physical laws.

Diffusion occurs where a dissolved substance which is present at higher concentration in one part of the solution than another spreads gradually until reaching an even distribution. The rate of diffusion is dependent upon the concentration difference between the various portions of the fluid, on temperature, fluid viscosity and particle size.

Osmosis takes place where different concentrations of a solute on either side of a membrane, which is permeable to the solvent but not the solute, cause the solvent to pass through the membrane in the direction which would equalise the concentrations. This process continues until the elevated solvent pressure equals the pressure of the solution — called the osmotic pressure.

Active transport is the process by which the cell actively expends energy to transport substances across the membrane. Since the substance concerned takes part in a pumping action,

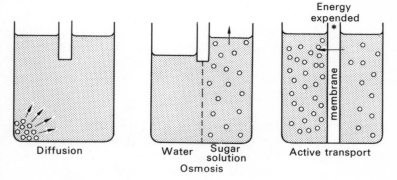

Fig. 1.2 Diffusion, osmosis and active transport

the machinery is referred to as a pump, e.g. the sodium pump transporting sodium ions.

These three systems are those concerned in exercise function, and are illustrated in Fig. 1.2.

Cell constituents

The basic constituents of a cell are protein, water, electrolytes, lipids and carbohydrates.

Protein   The basic building material of the cell is protein, forming 10–20 per cent of the cell weight. The structure, function and metabolism of the cell are dependent on the presence of certain proteins, one class of which, the enzymes, act as catalysts of chemical reactions in the cell. Proteins contain nitrogen, carbon, hydrogen, oxygen and sometimes sulphur. When hydrolysed (broken down by water) proteins split into simple nitrogen-containing molecules called amino acids. Those amino acids which cannot be manufactured in the human body but are obtained from other animal sources are called essential amino acids.

Water   Between 70 and 85 per cent of a cell is water, in which the cellular chemicals are either dissolved or suspended as particles.

Electrolytes   The major electrolytes are sodium, potassium, magnesium, phosphate, sulphate, bicarbonate and chloride ions. They are dissolved in the cellular water, provide inorganic chemicals for cell reactions, facilitate the transmission of electrical impulses and control some enzymatically-catalysed metabolic cell processes.

Lipids   Lipids are substances which are soluble in fat solvents. In the human, the lipids are neutral fat, phospholipids and cholesterol. Lipids are insoluble in water and, therefore, though present in only the low total concentration of 2–3 per cent, are ideally suited to form 40 per cent of the cellular membranes. Phospholipids are partly soluble in water and can selectively assist some substances to pass through membranes.

Carbohydrates   Amounting normally to only about 1 per cent of the cell mass, carbohydrates are major providers of energy for cell functioning. They are present in an insoluble form as glycogen, which is formed from glucose, the soluble and transportable form of usable carbohydrate.

Cell structures

The cell membrane is virtually a sandwich with outer layers of protein, and a filling of lipids. At intervals there are pores in the membrane which allow the passage of substances which are sufficiently small. The protein amounts to about 60 per

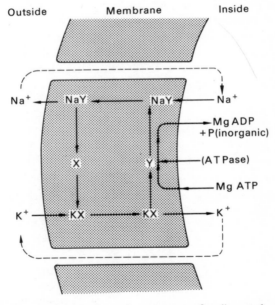

Fig. 1.3 Postulated mechanism for active transport of sodium and potassium through the cell membrane, showing coupling of the two transport mechanisms and delivery of energy to the system at the inner surface of the membrane

cent of the membrane, the remainder being mainly lipid. Of particular importance in sport is the stimulation of nerve and muscle cells, which depends on the transmission of sodium and potassium ions across the cell membrane. This is achieved by active transport, probably using a carrier substance, Fig. 1.3. We see that the maintenance of a high sodium ion concentration outside the cell (and potassium ion inside) is achieved in spite of a constant diffusion of these ions through the cell pores. The energy for the conversion of the carrier from sodium ion attractive to potassium ion attractive is obtained from processes within the cell.

The cytoplasm is a largely fluid medium containing mainly dissolved glucose, electrolytes and proteins, and also small quantities of lipids. The major organelles within the cytoplasm are the mitochondria and lysosomes.

Mitochondria   Depending on the normal energy usage level of the cell, mitochondria are present in numbers varying from a few hundred to a few thousand. They are the site for the formation of adenosine triphosphate (ATP), which is an

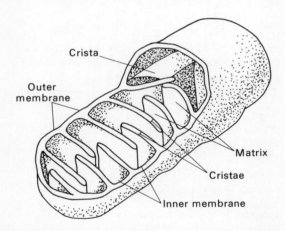

Fig. 1.4 Structure of a mitochondrion (redrawn from Robertson: *Biochem. Soc. Symp.* **16**, 38, Cambridge University Press, 1959)

energy-rich substance. The structure of a mitochondrion can be seen in Fig. 1.4. The inner matrix of the mitochondrion provides a series of storage areas termed cristae. These are the sites of oxidative enzymes and are where oxygen and fuels combine to create the basic energy source of the cell.

Lysosomes are the sites of cell 'digestion'. The lysosome is an aggregate of digestive enzymes, which operate on nutrients by hydrolysis – a process whereby a substance is split by water, one part of the substance combining with H and the other with OH (hydroxyl).

Certain specialised cells have special adaptations of these basic characteristics, or additional elements, which facilitate their particular function. Nerve cells, blood cells and muscle cells are described more fully in the chapters on their respective systems. Also of major importance in athletic function are secretory cells which form part of glands, and the secretory granules which are present both in secretory cells and in others such as nerve cells.

Cell energy

All cells have basically the same mechanisms of providing energy for their own functions: active transport, movement, chemical processes, etc. In sport the dominant function is movement, and the energy processes of the muscle cell will therefore be considered.

The most eminent of physiologists are still locked in fierce debate over the energy pathways in muscle, particularly at different levels, during different types of exercise, and under different environmental and dietary conditions. What follows is a simple account of the more commonly agreed mechanisms. Figure 1.5 shows the body system as an enclosed box, with oxygen and nutrients (carbohydrates, fats and proteins) entering, and carbon dioxide and urea leaving. The box is largely filled with a representation of a muscle cell, plus the liver as a storehouse of nutrients.

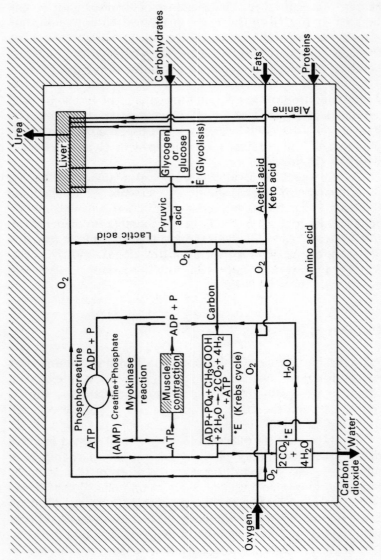

Fig. 1.5 Main energy routes of the body

Starting at the right of the figure, both fats and proteins may be converted into carbohydrate, and carbohydrate into fat, in the liver (gluconeogenesis and liponeogenesis respectively). The net result is to ensure an adequate supply of carbohydrate and fats to the muscle cell. The use of amino acids as fuel is negligible except during periods of extreme shortage of other sources of energy. Proteins can be used by direct oxidation to form water and carbon dioxide, providing energy (E) at that point, or they may be converted in the liver to fat or carbohydrate which then follows the usual energy pathway for those substances.

During many phases of submaximal work, fats are the preferred energy source of the muscle cell. They may enter the muscle cell either directly as acetic acid, or after conversion by the liver to keto acid. The carbohydrates, either as transportable glucose or as stored glycogen, split into molecules of pyruvic acid. This initial carbohydrate decomposition, because it requires no oxygen and yet releases energy, is said to be anaerobic.

The pyruvic, acetic and keto acids then follow the Krebs cycle, in which they combine with oxygen to provide the energy for the synthesis of the high energy compound adenosine triphosphate (ATP) from its constituents adenosine diphosphate (ADP) and phosphate (P). The end result is a quantity of ATP, plus hydrogen, which combines with oxygen to form water (thus releasing a little energy), and carbon dioxide.

That part of the pyruvic acid which is not immediately oxidised forms lactic acid, which then diffuses out of the cell. (Blood lactic acid may also diffuse back into the cell, but there appears to be no agreement among physiologists that the skeletal muscular cell utilises lactic acid as an energy source.) The pyruvic–lactic acid transformation is reversible when the lactic acid reaches a situation where there is a plentitude of oxygen.

The ATP which has been synthesised as a result of the energy released by these various processes is then available to release its energy to enable the cell to function. In so doing it is split down again to ADP + P. The oxidative reactions for resynthesis are relatively slow, and an immediate source of energy for the production of ATP can be provided instead by a reversible breakdown of phosphocreatine. The creatine and phosphate so formed are reconstituted later. In times of greater stress the muscle can also call on the myokinase reaction to split ADP further into adenosine monophosphate and P − another reversible operation. These latter two reactions may proceed without the presence of oxygen, and therefore contribute to the anaerobic function of the cell.

In addition to the nutrients, oxygen has to enter the body, taking part in oxidative actions both within and outside the cell. The end waste products of the system are mainly carbon dioxide which is exhaled, and a small amount of urea which is excreted. Another by-product is water, which enters the general fluid system of the body.

It appears as if a muscle cell can become exhausted, anaerobically by reaching a certain level of lactic acid within the cell, or aerobically by a gradual depletion of nutrient supply within the cell to zero. However, this is at present a hypothesis formulated from a wide variety of inconclusive evidence.

Cell equilibrium

The cell, in addition to having its own internal environment (intracellular fluid) is surrounded by the extracellular fluid. The basic composition of the two fluids can be seen in Fig. 1.6. The cell can live, operate and replicate for so long as some factors of its fluid environments are maintained within fine limits. Though the concentrations of some substances may vary enormously (e.g. glucose, lactic acid), others must be kept virtually unchanged. This is called *homeostasis* − the state of remaining unchanged, the law of constancy, the bedrock of human function.

The large difference in concentration across the cell membrane of the electrolytes maintains the electric potential and the permeability of the membrane. Chapter 6 describes how

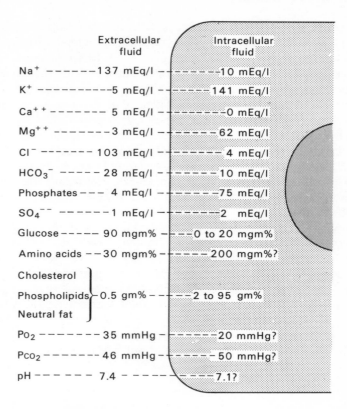

	Extracellular fluid		Intracellular fluid
Na^+	$-----137$ mEq/l	$-$	$------10$ mEq/l
K^+	$---------5$ mEq/l	$-$	$-----141$ mEq/l
Ca^{++}	$------$ 5 mEq/l	$-$	$------0$ mEq/l
Mg^{++}	$------3$ mEq/l	$-$	$-----62$ mEq/l
Cl^-	$------$ 103 mEq/l	$-$	$------$ 4 mEq/l
HCO_3^-	$-----28$ mEq/l	$-$	$-----10$ mEq/l
Phosphates	$---$ 4 mEq/l	$-$	$-----75$ mEq/l
SO_4^{--}	$------1$ mEq/l	$-$	$-----2$ mEq/l
Glucose	$-----$ 90 mgm%	$-$	$--0$ to 20 mgm%
Amino acids	$--30$ mgm%	$-$	$----200$ mgm%?
Cholesterol Phospholipids Neutral fat	-0.5 gm%	$--$	$--2$ to 95 gm%
Po_2	$-------35$ mmHg	$-$	$-----20$ mmHg?
Pco_2	$-------46$ mmHg	$-$	$-----50$ mmHg?
pH	$-----$ 7.4	$-----$	$---7.1?$

Fig. 1.6 Chemical compositions of extracellular and intracellular fluids

the potassium ion difference (gradient) maintains the potential of nerve cells (and a similar mechanism also applies to muscle cells). The calcium level of the extracellular fluid maintains the permeability of the cell membrane, and also is vitally concerned with the repair of damage to the membrane.

Acid–base balance

The concentration of hydrogen ions in the body fluids determines their acidity. Too high a concentration creates too acid a solution, too low, too basic a solution. The chemical functions of the cell depend greatly on the maintenance of the acid–base balance. The measured concentration is on a logarithmic scale having 7 as a neutral point, and normally registers 7·4 in the human (that is, slightly basic). The variation ranges only from 7·0 to 7·8, which may be approached in a sportsman when breath holding or when hyperventilating, because of the effects these activities have on extracellular carbon dioxide levels. Carbon dioxide combines with water to form carbonic acid (H_2CO_3), which is a weak acid and yet may still depress the pH value. Within the extracellular fluid are buffer substances, e.g. bicarbonate, and phosphate and protein, which maintain the acid–base balance within limits.

With so many transient changes occurring in the intra- and extracellular fluids, a continual and thorough mixing process is required. The osmotic, diffusion and active transport mechanisms bring into communication the intracellular fluid and the immediate extracellular fluid. Within the extracellular fluid there is constant diffusion and a passage of fluid constituents into the blood which then circulates through the body. This system is so effective that a virtually total mixing of all body fluids is achieved in about half an hour.

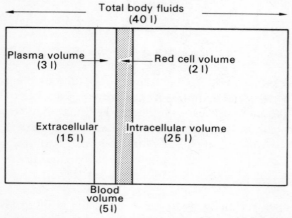

Fig. 1.7 Diagrammatic representation of the body fluids, showing the extracellular fluid volume, blood volume and total body fluids

The body fluids are as shown in Fig. 1.7. The plasma is similar in constitution to the other extracellular fluid, except in having a higher protein content. That part of the extracellular fluid which lies between the capillaries and the intracellular fluid is termed interstitial fluid. Some interstitial fluid (the lymph) flows in a network of vessels similar to the blood circulation. Lymphatic vessel walls are extremely permeable, and the system acts as an 'overflow' for the interstitial fluid, in addition to its important function in collecting and returning errant protein particles to the blood circulation.

Cell metabolism

The metabolic functions of the cell can be identified in terms of the use of energy. The process of breaking down nutrients from their original form into the simple end products releases energy, and is called catabolism. The process of building structural, storage and functional materials from simple constituents is called anabolism and consumes energy. The rate of energy usage of the cell is called its metabolic rate. The reference for the human is the basal metabolic rate (BMR), which is the energy consumed in maintaining life under standardised resting conditions (asleep if possible, at least 12 hours after the last meal) and under normal environmental conditions.

Metabolic rate is affected by many factors, and in the case of athletes principally by body temperature (positively), environmental temperature (negatively), digestion and exercise (positively) and excitement (positively). Of fundamental importance in the chemical activities of the cell is the temperature. Most cellular chemical reactions if performed in a test tube would require very high temperatures. The catalytic action of the cellular enzymes reduces the necessary temperature, and yet the reaction rates are increased if the cell temperature is raised, up to a maximum of approximately 40 °C. Beyond this point most cells lose their capacity to carry on metabolism, though some sportsmen have been observed to continue functioning at cellular temperatures in excess of 41 °C without ill effect.

External control

In addition to the 'self-regulating' or homeostatic controls of the cell, there are external agents affecting cellular function. Temperature has been discussed in the preceding paragraph. Chemical control is achieved by the action of hormones, a variety of substances with no uniform structural pattern. Hormones are secreted by the endocrine glands, and serve to control the function of certain specific groups of cells. The major hormones in exercise function are tabulated below.

Hormone	Gland	Cellular function controlled
Thyroxine	Thyroid	General cell metabolism
Adrenaline	Adrenal medulla	General cell metabolism
Noradrenaline	Adrenal medulla	General cell metabolism
Insulin	Pancreas	Carbohydrate utilisation
Adrenocortical	Adrenal cortex	Protein conversion to carbohydrate
Adrenalin	Adrenal cortex	Membrane permeability
Parathyroid	Parathyroids	Calcium balance

Cell function is also controlled by nerves, which relay electrical stimuli to the cell and release the control chemicals acetylcholine or noradrenaline. Acetylcholine is rapidly removed from the site of action by cholinesterase, which splits it into choline and acetic acid. Various drugs also affect cellular function, the more important being dealt with in Chapter 6.

CHAPTER TWO

Motility

All sportsmen move. Even the 'held' positions of gymnasts, divers, marksmen, etc. involve small fluctuations of movement. The sportsman's ability to move – against resistances, at speed, with precision, over long durations, under control – is fundamental to his sporting success. Movement can be caused by some external force, such as gravity or an opponent, but we are concerned with the movement the athlete produces in himself, or in some external object or implement. Such movement is caused mainly by muscular activity, though we should strictly include the movement of nervous impulses, which is electrochemical in nature.

It will help us if we consider muscular function as a whole, subdividing it later into motor, smooth, cardiac and ventilatory functions.

Muscle fibres

All muscle tissue is characterised by elongated cells having the property of contractility. The muscle fibres may vary in length from 3 mm to 50 cm, and are arranged in groups dependent upon their specific function (Fig. 2.1).

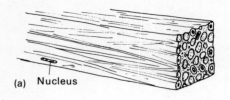

(a) Nucleus

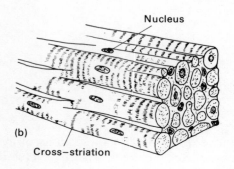

Nucleus

(b)

Cross–striation

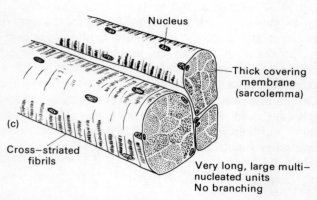

Nucleus

Thick covering
membrane
(sarcolemma)

(c)

Cross–striated
fibrils

Very long, large multi–
nucleated units
No branching

Fig. 2.1 (a) Smooth, unstriped visceral or involuntary muscle
(b) Cardiac or heart muscle
(c) Striated, striped, skeletal or voluntary muscle

Skeletal muscle function

The skeletal muscle belly is composed of perhaps thousands of individual muscle fibres, which blend into tendinous attachments at the extremities of the muscle. These fibres are brought into action upon receipt of a signal from a motor nerve (p. 26), which is transmitted via the neuromuscular junction, shown in Fig. 2.2.

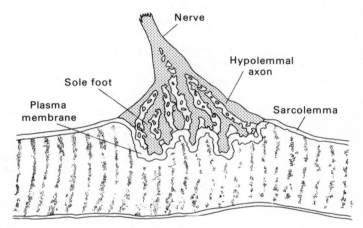

Fig. 2.2 The neuromuscular junction

The nerve fibre passes beneath the sarcolemna, and spreads into many branches. The total section is called a motor end plate. Each skeletal muscle may have between several hundred and several thousand motor nerve fibres, each innervating about 150 muscle fibres. All the muscle fibres innervated by one motor nerve are called units. These fibres are spread throughout the muscle, so that the function of one motor unit is not limited to a small area of the muscle. The proportion of end plates to muscle fibres is related to the degree of precise control required from each specific muscle. For example, muscles of the arm have a higher proportion of end plates than have leg muscles − and much greater precision of arm movement is possible than of leg movement.

The motor end plate branches have acetylcholine stored within them, which is released under the plasma membrane upon receipt of a minute nerve impulse. Acetylcholine increases the permeability of the membrane to sodium ions, which leak into the fibre and create an electrical potential at the end plate. When sufficiently large, the potential is transmitted as an action potential along the whole length of the fibre, in both directions from the end plate simultaneously. A further stored substance, cholinesterase, destroys the acetylcholine within approximately 5 milliseconds, thus cancelling the action potential and allowing the membrane to repolarise ready for the next nerve impulse. The system acts as a magnifier of the original nerve impulse, since the action potential is much greater in magnitude than the nerve potential. The speed of transmission of the action potential is approximately 5 metres per second, by comparison with the 50+ metres per second achieved by the large motor nerve fibres serving skeletal muscle.

We can see then that a skeletal muscle is served by motor nerve fibres, in motor units each serving perhaps many bundles of muscle fibres (Fig. 2.3). Each fibre may contain a thousand or more myofibrils arranged longitudinally, these

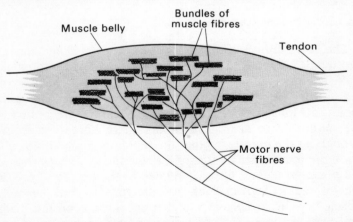

Fig. 2.3 A muscle, showing the distribution of nerve fibres supplying three motor units

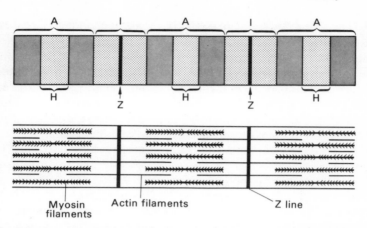

Fig. 2.4 *Above*: Schematic diagram of the light and dark areas in a myofibril
Below: Arrangement of the myosin and actin filaments in the sarcomeres

being composed of very many small filaments composed of actin or myosin (Fig. 2.4). The action potential travels not only along the surface of the fibre, but penetrates through the myofibrils, where it generates the release of calcium ions into the fluid surrounding the myofibrils *only for so long as* there

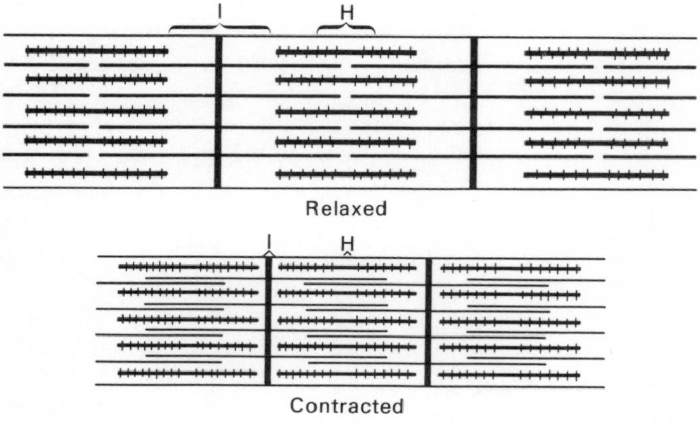

Relaxed

Contracted

Fig. 2.5 The relaxed and contracted states of a myofibril, showing sliding of the actin filaments into the channels between the myosin filaments

is an action potential present. If the action potential ceases, the release of calcium ions also ceases within a few milleseconds.

The calcium ions combine with myosin to form activated myosin which causes adenosine triphosphate (ATP) bonded to the actin filaments to release its stored energy (p. 21). This causes the actin and myosin filaments to interdigitate, thus shortening (or tending to shorten) the myofibril (Fig. 2.5).

Cardiac muscle function

Though cardiac muscle exhibits most of the characteristics of skeletal muscle, there are some most significant differences. The first of these is that cardiac muscle fibres are bound together in an interconnecting framework called a syncytium. One syncytium forms the walls and septum of the atria, the other syncytium forming the walls and septum of the ventricles. This interconnection is such that the stimulation of one fibre radiates through all the other fibres of that syncytium.

The second peculiarity of cardiac muscle is its inherent functional rhythm. The polarisation and depolarisation of the membrane tend to follow one another rhythmically without external nervous stimulation, at a rate in a normal human of approximately once every 800 milliseconds (72 per minute).

Lastly, cardiac muscle depolarisation lasts for 300 milliseconds, as against 2 milliseconds for skeletal muscles, thus maintaining the actin–myosin reaction for a sufficient time to enable the total cardiac musculature to complete a full blood ejection stroke (p. 74).

Smooth muscle function

The major difference of smooth muscle lies in the arrangement of its fibres, which are in two main groups. Firstly, internal organ (visceral) muscle fibres tend to interconnect in a syncytium similar to cardiac fibres. They tend therefore to function together whenever a stimulus is received by any single fibre. The second type is named multiunit smooth muscle, which has a separate fibre existence similar to skeletal muscle, but organised in an annular or tube-like structure. In this case more selective control is achieved by the facility of stimulating separate fibres. Multiunit fibres are found in blood vessels, and in constriction and dilation mechanisms such as the eye iris and various sphincters.

Visceral smooth muscle is inherently rhythmic in function, similar to cardiac muscle. The rate of contraction varies considerably according to the function of the organ concerned. Occasionally superimposed over visceral rhythmicity, and continually controlling multiunit muscle fibres, is the action of sympathetic and parasympathetic nerves of the autonomic nervous systems (p. 194). Sympathetic nerves cause the secretion of hormones called norepinephrine and epinephrine which stimulate some smooth fibres and inhibit others. Parasympathetic nerves secrete acetylcholine which in all cases has the opposite effect to the sympathetic hormones. The balance between these mechanisms controls each specific organ muscular function.

Gross movement

Since we are at present concerned with motility, we shall examine more closely the function of skeletal muscle.

It was thought for many years that a muscle fibre had a threshold stimulus level, above which it would contract with the maximum force of which it was at that time capable and below which it would not contract at all. This was called the all or nothing law, which has been called in question by some recent work.[43] However, what is certain is that there is always resistance to the movement of part or whole of the body. This might be due to the force of gravity for a high jumper, water resistance for a swimmer, internal structural resistances for the boxer's arm, opponents' mass in a rugby scrum – and so on. In order to cause movement, the musculature needs to call a sufficient number of sufficiently strong acting fibres into play to overcome the forces acting against it. The muscle fibres will receive motor nerve impulses in basically two ways, each achieving its end by a summation or integration of fibre function. The first method is to utilise a sufficient number of fibres, all acting maximally and simultaneously for a short period of time. This method is particularly used when a

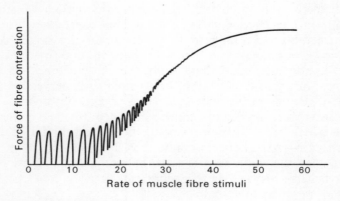

Fig. 2.6 Tetanisation of a muscle fibre

brief, powerful response is necessary. The second method is to re-stimulate each fibre while the previous contraction is still effective. Up to a rate of approximately 50 or 60 stimuli per second for most skeletal muscle, each stimulus adds a little more force to the previous one. At low rates of 10–20 stimuli per second the fibre contractions are discernible as separate pulses. Above this rate, the contractions blend together until reaching a smooth force development called tetanisation (Fig. 2.6).

Slower acting muscles, like postural muscles, tend to tetanise at a slower motor impulse rate, whereas faster acting muscles, such as manipulative muscles, tend to tetanise at 60 or more stimuli per second.

Speed of contraction

Skeletal muscle fibres exhibit one further characteristic which affects their function under a variety of sport conditions. Fibres can in fact be divided into 'quick contracting', or white fibres, and 'slow acting' or red fibres. Both types may be found in the same muscle, though the relative proportions depend upon the muscle's main function. Red muscles are generally slow contracting 'postural' muscles, white are fast action muscles. For example, the calf is composed of the soleus (a slow red postural muscle) and the gastrocnemius (a fast white propulsive muscle).

The speed with which a muscle can contract is dependent upon the type of resistance being overcome. With low resistances, the white fibres will dominate, at least in the early part of the movement; with high resistances, the red fibres will dominate. In either case, we are not really concerned with pure speed, but with acceleration, and the rate of acceleration is dependent upon the amount of force the muscle fibres can generate by comparison with the magnitude of the resistance, and upon the inherent contractile speed of the muscle fibres. Particularly in low resistance movements it has been discovered that speed of muscular contraction is more a function of neuromuscular coordination than of muscle strength.[31] The correlation between the static force a muscle is capable of exerting and the speed it is capable of generating is low at low resistances, but becomes greater as the resistance increases (and achieved speed decreases) reaching fairly high correlations in the region of 0.86.[79] In essentially low resistance movements, many other studies have shown there to be no significant relationship between static strength and the speed achievable by the limb.[10, 32, 69]

Force of contraction

Broadly speaking, the strength of muscular contraction is dependent upon, firstly, the amount of muscle tissue available and, secondly, how much of it is used. It has long been known that bigger muscles are stronger,[73] and that this size is due both to an expansion of the myofibrils and an increase in the number of effective fibres. Accompanying the structural enlargement, there is an increase in the capacity of the muscle to store nutrients, and in the blood supply to the muscle.

Of greatest importance in muscular force production is the selection and deployment of fibres. The control methods involved will be discussed at a later stage (Chapter 6) but it can be stated with a fair degree of certainty that a sportsman is never able to call into play *all* the fibres of a given muscle. Great improvements in strength have been recorded from subjects under hypnosis and other psychological procedures.[41]

Muscle endurance

We have seen that the energy for muscle contraction is obtained by splitting the high energy compound ATP. Adenosine diphosphate (ADP) and phosphate formed by this process are reconverted to ATP by energy released either anaerobically, mainly by the breakdown of stored glycogen to lactic acid, or aerobically by oxidation of carbohydrates and fat. There is evidence that no oxidation of proteins takes place during muscle work.[54] If muscle endurance is defined as the ability to undertake repeated contractions over a period of time, then it can be seen that the limits to endurance are set by:

(1) the store of glycogen within the muscle mitochondria;
(2) the supply of carbohydrates and fats and oxygen to the muscle during contractions;
(3) the ability of the motor nerves to repeatedly stimulate the muscle.

Since the initial contraction of a muscle fibre is anaerobic, the achievement of aerobic muscle work (and the delay or prevention of accumulation of fatigue products) requires some relaxation of the fibre. In fact, muscle fibres work most efficiently in terms of endurance when contraction and relaxation alternate with a sufficiently long relaxation period to clear the lactic acid between contractions. Endurance is achieved by rotating the work load around different motor units, allowing some to relax while others work.[28, 57, 74]

Most recent studies demonstrate that within this macro-function of muscle there is a sharp differentiation between the metabolisms of red and white fibres; and, therefore, a differentiation in their functions. In all fibres, the activity of glycolysis (anaerobic fibres) is inversely proportional to the oxidative and lipid mechanisms, either one or the other predominating. Fibres may therefore be termed glycolytic or oxidative. The glycolytic fibres (white) are relatively poorly capillarised, are suitable for sudden relatively isolated contractions, and fatigue quite quickly. They merely need to replace glycogen and remove lactic acid after their activity.

Oxidative (red) fibres, on the other hand, are well supplied with capillaries in order to maintain repeated contractions by continually replenishing oxygen and fuel during activity.

Anaerobic muscle function

Current sports terminology has tended to use the terms aerobic and anaerobic to describe levels of work load relative to the maximum oxygen intake of the individual, since that determines the rate of 'combustion of fuels' in the total body. However, a more accurate definition recognises that the breakdown of ATP to ADP + P proceeds without oxygen – therefore all work is anaerobic in that sense, and anaerobic work is defined as *the splitting of glycogen and high energy phosphates in the muscle cell*. Short periods of intensely high activity, such as weightlifting or sprint running, may proceed under virtually completely anaerobic conditions. A duration of $2\frac{1}{2}$ to 3 minutes is sufficient to reduce local muscle ATP to a level where the muscle is exhausted. In order to maintain contractions it is necessary continually to replenish the ATP, which is done by stored muscle glycogen during high intensity work, and an insufficiently large store could be a limit to anaerobic work.[4, 5]

High lactate values are commonly observed in blood during exercise of various durations and intensities, but in some instances even exhaustive effort fails to raise blood lactate above resting levels, and prolonged severe exercise may even result in low blood lactate concentration.[72] However, the blood lactate level is not always a good indicator of muscle lactate concentration, and no studies have revealed that lactate accumulation in the muscle is a limiting factor *per se*.

It has been suggested that blood pH is a limiting factor in anaerobic work,[8] but unpublished observations of Hermansen and Wadell suggest that the hypothesis is ill founded and, moreover, that intracellular pH was not demonstrably a limiting factor either.

Oxygen debt

The maximum oxygen uptake of an individual athlete determines the level of aerobic energy output of which he is capable. When working in excess of these levels, other biochemical changes produce the necessary energy, these changes

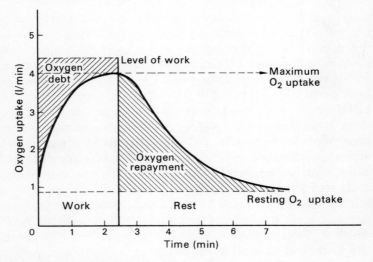

Fig. 2.7 Oxygen uptake during anaerobic work

being reversible later when oxygen uptake can remain temporarily in excess of a lowering in energy expenditure (Fig. 2.7).

In this instance work has been at a very high rate for the total work time, as in an 800 m track race. The respiratory adjustments to the exercise are not instantaneous, and by the time that maximal oxygen uptake is reached, an *oxygen debt* has accumulated. While at maximal oxygen uptake, which is still lower than the real requirement for oxygen, further debt accrues until the end of exercise. During recovery, the oxygen uptake remains in excess of resting requirements until the debt is cleared, the rate of repayment dropping off very rapidly over the first few minutes and then returning more gradually to normal over a much longer time – perhaps an hour or more.

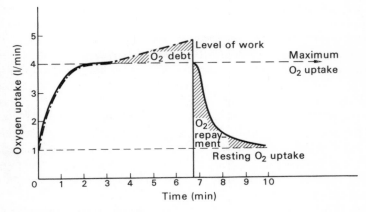

Fig. 2.8 Oxygen uptake during mixed work

If the rate of work can be nicely adjusted to match the maximum acceleration of oxygen uptake, until passing the level of maximum oxygen uptake, then the tolerable oxygen debt will allow an increase in the total work done (Fig. 2.8). If the work is all performed at a high but submaximal oxygen uptake level continuously, an oxygen debt will occur during the first phase of work which can be repaid during the later work phase (Fig. 2.7). This phenomenon occurs during longer distance events, with the initial lag in respiratory response falling behind the demands of the fast start, and may also occur during tactical bursts during the race.

Anaerobic work capacity

Whatever is the limiting element in anaerobic work — and we have seen that a reduction in the concentration of ATP coupled with a disappearance of its immediate resynthesising agent, phosphocreatine, is probably the major limiting element — the capacity of the individual sportsman to endure a large oxygen debt is of major importance in short-duration endurance. This is best seen in events such as long sprints, middle distance and short parts of long distance locomotion competition (walking, running, swimming, cycling, rowing, canoeing, etc.). There is direct evidence that oxygen debt capacity is related to maximum work ability in sportsmen.[34]

There is also a capacity for anaerobic work which is not of the same order of magnitude as maximum oxygen debt. Indeed, if the maximum oxygen debt is seen as a summation of the ATP exhaustion in every skeletal muscle cell, it is unlikely that that level can ever be reached by an athlete. Therefore, the limit is reached in a critical muscle group which, if sufficiently gross (as in locomotion muscle groups), will have consumed a large amount of energy in the process — and hence a large oxygen debt. If work is limited to a small muscle group, then the limit to anaerobic work is still set by the ATP availability but the amount of energy consumed before 'exhaustion' is reached may be relatively small. This phenomenon has been observed during heavy forearm work with the blood supply occluded.[7]

Aerobic muscle function

Although human muscle tissue can subsist anaerobically for relatively short periods of time, and each individual contraction can be viewed as basically an anaerobic incident, the great majority of the cellular functions must be considered as aerobic. The muscular system can be seen as an engine, converting biochemically borne energy from one source (brought by the blood) into the production of force for work, and eliminating the biochemical byproducts of the system. The continuing and limiting requirements for aerobic muscle function are oxygen, and energy carriers such as pyruvic, acetic and keto acids. The limit of the sportsman's ability to work aerobically depends then upon his nutrient supply mechanism (storage – both local and central – and transport) and his oxygen supply mechanism. It may also depend on his carbon dioxide and lactate clearance mechanisms, though this is less clear. All these parameters will be discussed later.

This limit has tended to be measured in performance tests by the maximal oxygen uptake, and by the blood glucose, free fatty acid and muscle glycogen levels. By far the easiest and most common parameter to measure has been maximum oxygen uptake (V_{O_2}), either by direct or indirect methods,[1] and this parameter has been shown to correlate highly with athletic ability by many workers. Blood and muscle lactate levels have not been shown to relate consistently to maximal aerobic function.

Total muscle endurance

Except in cases where a short duration high activity level response is necessary, an athlete's muscles operate most efficiently in an aerobic state. If the total energy production is required to be high, then the muscles should perform at or near their maximum aerobic level for as much of the time as possible, with as few excursions into anaerobia as are compatible with tactical considerations. Such excursions should be followed by a depression of work rate sufficient to allow the reversion of intramuscular anaerobic effects, except in the case of 'terminal sprints' where recovery can be made at leisure.

Cardiac muscle function

The heart muscle fibres behave in a very similar way to skeletal muscle. There are, however, some important differences.

Refractory period

Throughout the total period of contraction, heart muscle fibres are absolutely refractory. They are incapable of the tetanising effect achievable by skeletal muscle. This period is necessary to allow one contraction to be completed and recovered from before another is initiated. The absolute refractory period for cardiac muscle is about 0·2 seconds at normal resting rates.

Metabolism

Cardiac muscle fibres cannot function after their oxygen supply has been exhausted. They have not, therefore, the same capacity as skeletal muscle to incur an oxygen debt. There is however evidence that cardiac muscle cells are capable of taking up lactate as well as glucose from the blood.[81]

Impulse transmission

Whereas skeletal muscle fibres transmit action potentials at approximately 5 metres per second, only the specialised cardiac Purkinje fibres compare at 4 m/sec, with transmission in the atrial walls much slower (1 m/sec) and in the atrio/ventricular node as low as 0·2 m/sec. This is compatible with the slower contraction and the 'squeezing out' effect necessary in the heart.

The working muscle

Muscle tissues are the physical force-producing agents of the body. They produce, tend to produce or control movement of the body. The ways in which they do this have been classified under three forms of action, and their ability to function differs from one to another type of action.

Firstly, muscles exerting force can be actually shortening, that is, the extremities of the muscle become closer together. This is called *concentric* muscle work.

Secondly, muscles exerting force (i.e. tending to contract) can be actually lengthening, that is, the muscle extremities are being pulled apart by some force greater than that produced by the muscle. This is called *eccentric* muscle work.

Lastly, muscles exerting force (i.e. tending to contract) may remain stationary, that is, the muscle neither lengthens nor shortens because its force is matched by some balancing force acting in the opposite direction. This is called *static* muscle work.

Concentric and eccentric work are commonly said to be isotonic, a quite misleading term since the moving muscles do not exhibit a constancy of tone, tension or force. However, the term is used mainly to differentiate between these two actions and static work, which is called isometric – a more logical term.

During the 1960s, developments in resistance training methods have disclosed an adapted form of isotonic work which is called isokinetic. Such work occurs when a muscle moves concentrically or eccentrically, exerting the maximum contraction force of which it is capable at each stage of the movement. Whereas normally during isotonic work the force exertable by the muscle is limited to its maximum during the least mechanically efficient part of the movement (the sticking point), during isokinetic work the muscle is exerting greater forces during the mechanically more efficient parts of the movement.

If one considers that the energy production in the muscle cell tends to cause the actin and myosin filaments to inter-digitate 'concentrically', then eccentric work (and to a lesser extent static work) can be seen to cause a breakdown in the tendency bonds between the filaments. Certainly, muscles are incapable of exerting as much force or endurance during eccentric work, and residual soreness and trauma are more often experienced in muscles during and after eccentric work of many different types.

The greatest force can be exerted by a muscle when it is acting isometrically. It should be borne in mind that:

(a) *absolutely* static muscle function is non-existent in sport;
(b) even when the muscle extremities are fixed, the elastic properties of individual fibres ensure that rotation of contractions between various motor units creates shortening and lengthening of the fibres.

It can be seen, therefore, that no muscle function in sport is truly isometric. However, for most purposes 'held' positions and *extremely* slow movements are considered as isometric.

The classical equation governing force and velocity of human muscle is

$$V = b(P_0 - P)/(P + a)$$

where V = initial velocity of shortening, P = actual force acting on the muscle, P_0 = the maximal force which the muscle can develop, a represents a force constant and b represents a velocity constant. This rather simple equation is of the type which allows the b/a relationship to provide a limiting value to muscle velocity (i.e. a muscle behaves as a damped elastic body), and yet shows force to tend to a maximum as velocity tends to zero.

Comparisons of endurance between isometric and isotonic work are somewhat nebulous in view of the difficulty of achieving true isometric muscle fibre contraction. On the other hand, it has been demonstrated that recovery is much faster after isometric work.[11]

Muscle training

In a text of this nature it is necessary to examine closely the effects of different types of training on skeletal and cardiac musculature. Little is known of the effects of training on smooth muscle, but it seems logical to expect similar changes in that tissue also. To the athlete, training is seen as a planned approach to the improvement of function. That this concept should be applied to smooth muscle is not unreasonable but since smooth muscle is controlled through the autonomic nervous system, any attempt to adapt or stress smooth muscle function has to be indirect.

Skeletal muscle

Training of skeletal muscle can be divided into several main categories:

(1) strength – the ability to exert force;
(2) velocity – the ability to contract quickly;
(3) power – the ability to perform much work in little time;
(4) endurance – the ability to maintain contractions (a) aerobically and (b) anaerobically;
(5) flexibility – the ability to be stretched without damage.

Strength

Earlier in this chapter we saw that strength was dependent on muscle size and fibre deployment. In the total body situation this has been demonstrated for animals in general,[36] and by many studies in human populations. The concept of muscularity being dependent on basic body structure was clearly enunciated by Sheldon,[67] and has been reinforced by many other workers. Muscular individuals are stronger than others, and that strength is an important attribute in sports in general has been demonstrated frequently.[13, 80]

In 1933 there was a significant review by Steinhaus[73] of a number of reports which established the modern belief that overload training causes hypertrophy of latent or relatively latent muscle fibres, giving increased size and strength. There is also a more recent discovery that training can cause an increase in the total number of myofibrils.[27] The majority of strength training systems impose a progressively increasing resistance to muscle contraction, using a level of resistance which permits very few repetitions of contraction before exhaustion.

The appearance of a report from Hettinger and Muller [35] in 1953 caused a world-wide disturbance of these views, since these authors reported large strength gains (5 per cent per week) accruing from isometric training at low activity levels (e.g. 1/3 maximum force) held for only a matter of seconds each day. A vogue for isometric training was initiated which has lasted to the present time, accompanied by a great number of studies which appeared either to confirm or contradict the original findings, reviewed by Rasch [59] and re-evaluated by Royce. [64] The difficulty lay in the fact that the original research had been performed on subjects of low strength, and such great gains could not be achieved in trained athletes. Royce's work indicated that the rate of gain in static strength from isometric training lay on a decreasing curve, with an asymptote representing a theoretical maximum termed *Endkraft*. It is of interest that the isometric training effect was expressed in terms of static strength, since strength training tends to produce maximal effects specifically in the positions and types (static or dynamic) of effort made.

Velocity

The inherent velocity of contraction exhibited by a muscle fibre can best be expressed as the relation between the time taken from the receipt of an action signal at the neuromuscular junction to the eventual contraction of that fibre and the total distance of shortening of the fibre. This parameter is understandably difficult to measure in the intact sportsman, and we have seen that part of the time is consumed by the propagation of the action potential along the muscle fibre (at about 5 m/sec). It is not known if training can improve this function, but it ought to be realised that in a fibre of (say) 10 cm length, this transmission time would amount to only 0·02 sec. Laboratory studies of muscle function have been performed in which a single instantaneous stimulus is applied to a motor nerve. The duration of the resulting contraction can vary between 0·1 and 0·003 sec, and is called a twitch. Figure 2.9 shows the different durations of contractions of several muscle twitches.

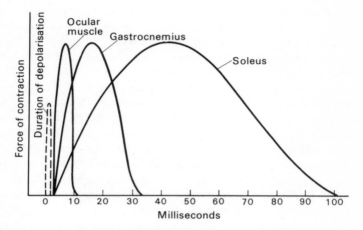

Fig. 2.9 Isometric muscle twitches of ocular, gastrocnemius and soleus muscles, illustrating the different durations of contraction

It can be seen that depolarisation time in these studies is approximately 2 msec, followed by contraction times of 7, 29 and 97 msec for different muscles. The precise effects of training in these cases is not known.

Power

The velocity of muscle contraction in its pure sense is difficult to study, but the product of velocity and force is power, and the power of muscular contraction can be more easily investigated *in vivo* since the internal and external resistances to movement can form a part of the investigation. Most studies of power have been of gross musculature, which forms the basis of most sports movements. The most widely used tests have been of standing jump distances, both horizontal and vertical. These have been shown to be related to each other by many workers, Fleishman [24] reporting a correlation of 0·60 between the two, and Thomas achieving 0·673 in his study of several hundred international sportsmen – also demonstrating lower but significant correlations between these power tests and a wide variety of static muscular force measures. [75]

Other studies have shown very low or zero correlations between jump power and anthropometric variables, [14, 68] but there are indications that power measures may correlate with sports ability. [13]

More sophisticated biomechanical analyses of muscular movement have examined the relationships between power, strength, muscle mass, body segment mass and speed. [10, 31, 32, 33, 69] It is apparent from these that muscle power is not highly correlated with other variables, and that the major component of an individual athlete's power is some unique capacity other than 'these parameters. Henry has postulated that manifestations of power such as jump tests are conditioned by quite specific motor coordination elements. [30] Much research remains to be performed before these relationships are fully understood.

Increases in effective muscle power, therefore, would seem to be achievable by improving the neuromuscular coordination of the motor units responsible for a specific movement, and by increasing the *dynamic* force of the musculature concerned. There is a general acceptance of dynamic training methods throughout sport, reviewed by Berger [3] and Hooks. [38] Experimental evidence to support the dynamic force development component is provided by several authors [9, 10, 56, 70] but there is less conclusive information concerning neuromuscular coordination, which will be treated in more detail later.

Endurance

In 1954 Henry examined locomotor speed and oxygen requirements during sprinting over various distances. [29] His mathematical model of the results demonstrated that, after a short period required to reach maximum velocity, there was an immediate decrease in performance. This decrease could be characterised by an exponential curve, with an initial sharp drop gradually levelling out to a steady state. This work was soon followed by a number of studies by Clarke[12] which demonstrated that increased muscle endurance was related to increased muscle strength, to the optimal work position of each muscle and to the cadence of the activity.

There is general agreement that muscle endurance may be developed by exercises of a multi-repetitive nature, and that this improvement can be due in part to alterations in the sequential use of locomotor musculature[15, 28] which is a learned muscular skill. Apart from the increased stores of nutrients accompanying hypertrophic increase through training, an important study using muscle biopsy techniques performed by Saltin[65] showed that the precompetitive training phase could be adjusted to produce a great augmentation of the muscle glycogen stores. This was demonstrated to give increased muscle endurance, and was achieved by an alternation of rest and exhaustion training, and of low and high carbohydrate ingestion. The effects of this training routine were temporary but significant. Similar endurance effects have been demonstrated over a wide range of exercise modes by the use of carbohydrate supplements alone.[76, 77]

There is a hypothesis that repeated stimulation of the motor nerve can result in fatigue at the neuromuscular junction. There appears to be no clear evidence that this phenomenon is a limiting factor in muscle endurance, or that such an event could be avoided by correct training. Indeed, Merton's study of muscle action potential and muscle tension demonstrated that for maximal voluntary muscular contractions there was no evidence that fatigue was due to deterioration of the action potential—contraction coupling.[52]

Many of the problems concerning effects of training on muscle endurance remain to be solved, but advances in muscle biopsy technique will no doubt allow this development in the near future. Most research so far has been undertaken on laboratory animals, particularly rats. Apart from any other dissimilarities which there may be between this species and the athlete, there is great difficulty in controlling the relative exercise levels of such animals, and findings are occasionally contradictory. However, there is a degree of agreement that strenuous training for some months leads to an increase in size and number of mitochondria in rat skeletal muscle. The same effect was not achieved during light training of a slightly shorter duration.[25, 37]

The capacity for anaerobic metabolism has been shown to improve in the human as a result of a long period of training, using blood lactate level as the parameter.[34] Figure 2.10 shows typical lactate data during training.

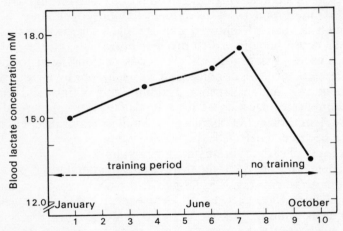

Fig. 2.10 Blood lactate concentration (peak value) after maximal exercise (100 m swimming) during the training period and after $2\frac{1}{2}$ months with no training

In summary, it can be stated that muscle endurance can be developed with training by:

(1) an increase in strength;
(2) a development of neuromuscular coordination;
(3) improved cadence selection;

(4) increased muscle glycogen stores;
(5) increased muscle mitochondrial fraction;
(6) increased lactate production.

There are probably other effects, particularly with regard to the development of ATP and phosphocreatine stores through training.

Flexibility

Muscle fibre has elastic properties; it is capable of being stretched. In fact, when the body is in the anatomical position, all skeletal muscles are under a certain degree of stretch, since their 'natural' length is shorter than that required. When a sportsman is unfortunate enough to suffer a snapped Achilles tendon the muscle returns to its natural length with the end of the severed tendon several inches up the calf, and the musculature unusually bunched up. Additionally, skeletal muscles are constantly in receipt of a low level of motor nerve impulses, maintaining a small degree of tension which is called tone. These two factors are interconnected, since muscle which is stretched is reflexly stimulated to contract. The mechanisms of this control system will be discussed later. At this stage, it is important to view the muscle as a two-component system, the contractile part of the system running *in series* with the connective tissue which is more or less elastic (including tendon which has only slight elasticity).

The length to which a muscle is stretched before contraction has an effect on the strength of contraction (Fig. 2.11). The optimal length of muscle in the sportsman for maximal force production coincides almost exactly with its maximal position of stretch (but because of the alteration of the mechanical efficiency of the joint–lever system of that muscle, the same may not hold true for the *effective* force production over the joint).

Flexibility in the sportsman is generally defined as the

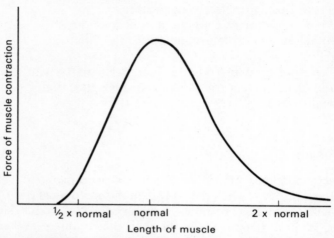

Fig. 2.11 Effect of the initial length of a muscle on the contractile force developed
following muscle excitation

extent of movement about a joint, from a position of maximum extension to one of maximum flexion. The limits in
extension are commonly set by:

(1) degree of relaxation in flexor muscles;
(2) length of flexor muscles;
(3) length of ligaments binding the joint;
(4) skeletal structure.

The limits in flexion are similar except that it is the flexibility of the extension muscles which pertains. It may be
added that in some cases, the limit to a particular movement
may be set by none of these factors – for example, the limit to
hip flexion with knee bent may be determined by the prox-
imity of the trunk.

It has been shown that systematic heavy resistance exercises for strength need not reduce muscle flexibility.[50] Reduc-
tions in flexibility *may* occur, but this is seen as a defect in the
training method, associated with a failure to take powerful
joint movements to their extreme. Some of the strongest

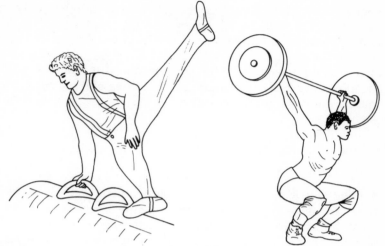

Fig. 2.12 Flexibility in gymnastics and weightlifting

sportsmen, particularly gymnasts and weightlifters, are also extremely flexible (Fig. 2.12).

Conversely, exercises which strengthen muscles are very commonly seen to result in increased muscle flexibility.[20, 44, 46] Very little is known about the mechanisms underlying this training effect. Possible causes are:

(1) an elongation of muscle connective tissue;
(2) a relaxation of muscle contractive tissue tone;
(3) an increase in force production by antagonist musculature;
(4) an increase in basic elasticity of the muscle tissue.

If stretching exercises are to be performed with the specific intention of increasing muscle flexibility, the stretch positions should proceed slightly beyond the point of comfort.[6, 49]

Historically, fashion in Physical Education has provided several methods of training muscle flexibility. Ballistic stretching, which generates body segment momentum which is eventually overcome by the limits of the movement is advocated by some,[6, 49] but contraindicated for its 'muscle straining' effect by others.[71, 78] Passive stretching has its proponents [45, 49, 78] and opponents.[26, 71] Rhythmic active stretching as described by Rathbone [60] is most commonly favoured for its relaxation effect on antagonist muscles, its 'self control' function and the allowance it makes for gradual loosening and recovery of muscle fibres during the exercise.

Factors affecting muscle function

Temperature

Studies of effects of altering muscle temperature have been relatively few. The actual temperature in a muscle may be quite different from the surface skin temperature in the same area,[23] making it necessary for heat sensitive devices to be inserted into the muscle, or for inferential measures to be made from other parameters such as blood flow. It has for many years been considered that elevated muscle temperature results in improved performance, primarily because the higher levels of muscular activity are accompanied by great heat production. However, it is probably more rational to consider the heat produced during muscle work to be an effect of metabolic inefficiency, than a cause of work efficiency.

The rise in temperature of a muscle upon receipt of an action potential is quite rapid. A. V. Hill's long series of investigations demonstrated that there is an immediate rise in temperature with the receipt of the nervous stimulus which actually precedes the beginning of contraction (Fig. 2.13).

The heat production associated with the activity can be described as initial heat, most of which is a reflection of the energy production in maintaining the active state (activation heat). During isometric activity virtually all the heat is activation heat. During concentric isotonic work, there is an extra amount of heat production called *shortening heat*, which is proportional to the amount of shortening of the muscle. If the muscle performs work during its recovery to initial length,

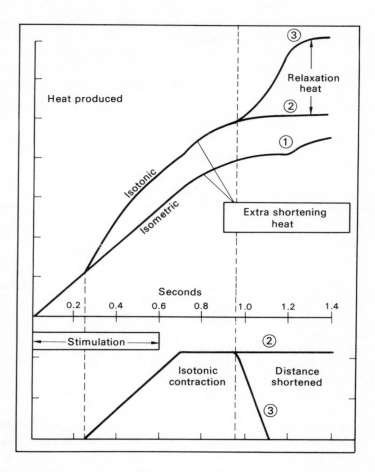

Fig. 2.13 Heat production in isometric and isotonic contractions. 1, 2 and 3 show
heat production associated with tetanus produced by 0·6 sec stimulation of an isolated muscle at 0° C.
(1) Isometric, no mechanical work done
(2) Isometric up to dotted line, then isotonic. Weight supported during
relaxation, hence no relaxation heat
(3) As 2, but the weight is not supported during relaxation. The work
done by the muscle during this relaxation appears as relaxation heat
Below the line scale are shown the corresponding mechanical records
(from results by A. V. Hill)

there is further heat production which has been less logically named by Hill as relaxation heat.

Following muscle activity there is a further production of heat, recovery heat, which is associated with the metabolic recovery of the muscle cells. This is approximately equal to the initial heat:

$$\text{initial heat} \begin{cases} \text{activation} \\ \text{shortening} \\ \text{relaxation} \end{cases} \text{heat} \simeq \text{recovery heat}$$

Activation and recovery heat arise from chemical processes liberating energy inefficiently (human musculature is approximately 25 per cent efficient when working optimally). Shortening heat and relaxation heat are due to physical processes during movement.

The bulk of the work establishing the foregoing information has been performed on isolated animal muscle fibres in the laboratory. Recent advances in the use of thermocouples have permitted the human to be studied while working. Direct observations on working muscles have provided long awaited data,[61] which force a reconsideration of all previous examinations of sports performance based on the hypothesis that surface and core temperatures provide adequate indications of muscle temperature. In particular, it has been demonstrated that the working muscle temperature is much greater than the rectal temperature, even at submaximal loads.[66] The difference between the two is proportional to the ratio between the metabolic rate and the maximal metabolic rate, which if extrapolated to maximal work levels would mean even higher muscle temperatures than the core temperatures of 41·1 °C recorded on marathon runners.[58]

The specific action of heat on the muscle fibre is probably best described as a process for facilitating metabolic function (the heat acting as a catalyst in the chemical reactions), and also as a method of diminishing the perceived pain of some forceful or prolonged work (heat acting as an analgesic).[23]

Cramps and soreness

Cramp is a frequent and occasionally critical phenomenon in sports performance. Even though the difficulties of investigating cramp are very great, a certain amount of experimentation has been performed. In particular, electromyographic studies have shown cramp to be a disturbance of the threshold level of action potential transmission in the muscle. Instead of motor units firing asynchronously, nearly all units fire simultaneously and at greatly increased frequencies (up to 300/sec). This results in a painful spasm of the muscle, with an excessive contraction of the fibres and a 'balling' of the muscle belly.[17, 18, 48]

The most common cause of cramp in sport is a disturbance in the body electrolyte and fluid balance, through profuse sweating and unbalanced fluid and electrolyte intake. This system will be described later. In some way not fully understood, this imbalance affects the level of excitability of the motor units. Certainly, the cramp may be relieved by a gradual stretching of the affected muscle,[55] but it is likely to return if the muscle fibres are contracted again.

The eminent American worker, De Vries, has performed many experiments in this area and has postulated a theory of muscular cramp and soreness based in part on observations of typical fatigue curves of exercised muscles stimulated repetitively:

(1) exercise causes ischaemia in the active muscle;[2, 62]
(2) ischaemia causes pain;
(3) the pain brings about a reflex tonic muscle contraction;[55]
(4) the tonic contraction causes further ischaemia.

It can be seen that this constitutes a vicious circle, resulting in a severe contracture.

De Vries's carefully considered development of a system of relief of cramps and soreness by static stretching [19, 20] was based upon the following rationale:

(1) it appears that there are two components to the muscle spindle reflex: phasic and static;[53]

(2) the phasic response is proportional to the muscle stretching, both in magnitude and rate; [53]

(3) the tendon reflex receptors have a higher threshold, but when they are stimulated they cause a reflex relaxation of the whole muscle; [51]

(4) steady stretching depresses the stretch reflex response; [40]

(5) the amplitude of the action potentials decreases in large human muscles when they are stretched, [42] which phenomenon is related to tendon receptor activity. [47]

De Vries's theory is an attractive one, especially since his wide observations suggest that soreness due to ruptured muscle fibres is far less frequent than had commonly been supposed. [39] Nor does he attribute muscle cramp and soreness to a residual high lactic acid level, though this biochemical possibility should not be divorced from De Vries's neuromuscular reasoning. It is common practice to use heat and massage in the treatment of muscular soreness, the aim being to clear residual waste products by increased blood flow. That this is effective may be taken as an indication that the biochemical hypothesis may be valid. It would seem that both stretching and circulation stimulants have their part to play in the relief of muscle cramp and soreness.

Experiments in muscle function

Since the function of the cardiac muscle will be considered later, experiments will be limited to skeletal muscle at this stage.

Referring to the Appendix for a note on suitable experiment construction, the student is advised that the parameters may be divided into the following suitable subgroups. These are *in vivo* experiments, which may be supplemented by laboratory experiments with isolated muscle preparations. One or more items from each group may be examined in one experiment, with all groups being investigated or one or more groups held constant during the experiment.

Physical dimension:

- (a) one muscle group *v* another muscle group;
- (b) one subject's muscle group *v* the same group in another subject;
- (c) one muscle before and after training hypertrophy;
- (d) subjects of one body type *v* subjects of another body type.

Work condition:

- (a) temperature, either externally applied or internally generated;
- (b) degree of stretch;
- (c) degree of fatigue;
- (d) presence of tremor;
- (e) motivation;
- (f) energy storage (starved, high carbohydrate diet, etc.);
- (g) electrolyte balance (sweating, with fluid replacement but no salt).

Work type:

- (a) static, eccentric or concentric;
- (b) degree of effort (maximal, or set proportion of maximal);
- (c) aerobic or anaerobic (including circulatory occlusion);
- (d) cadence (rate and length of repetitions);
- (e) passive or actively induced movements.

Muscle function:

- (a) against resistance — bodyweight, deadweight, springs, dynamometer;
- (b) frequency and amplitude of electromyogram trace;
- (c) velocity of body segment moved;
- (d) flexibility (measured at joint, or by muscle length);
- (e) power (work done per time taken).

References

1. ASTRAND, P-O (1954) 'A nomogram for calculation of aerobic capacity (physical fitness) from pulse rate during sub-maximal work'. *Journal of Applied Physiology*, **7**, 218.
2. BARCROFT, H. and MILLEN, J. L. E. (1939) 'The blood flow through muscle during sustained contraction'. *Journal of Physiology*, **97**, 17.
3. BERGER, R. A. (1963) 'Effects of dynamic and static training on vertical jumping ability'. *Research Quarterly of the American Association for Health, Physical Education and Recreation*, **34**, 419.
4. BERGSTROM, J. and HULTMAN, E. (1967) 'A study of the glycogen metabolism during exercise in man'. *Scandinavian Journal of Clinical and Laboratory Investigation*, **19**.
5. BERGSTROM, J., HERMANSEN, L., HULTMAN, E. and SALTIN, B. (1967) 'Diet, muscle glycogen and physical performance'. *Acta physiologica scandinavica*, **71**.
6. BILLIG, H. E. and LOENWENDAHL, E. (1949) *Mobilisation of the human body*. Stanford University Press: Stanford, Calif.
7. BROOKE, J. D. and THOMAS, V. Unpublished observations.
8. CERETELLI, P. (1967) 'Lactacid oxygen debt in acute and chronic hypoxia'. In, *Exercise at altitude*. Exerpta Medica Foundation: Milan.
9. CHUI, E. F. (1964) 'Effects of isometric and dynamic weight training exercises upon strength and speed of movement'. *Research Quarterly of the American Association for Health, Physical Education and Recreation*, **35**, 246.
10. CLARKE, D. H. and HENRY, F. M. (1961) 'Neuromotor specificity and increased speed from strength development'. *Research Quarterly of the American Association for Health, Physical Education and Recreation*, **32**, 315.
11. CLARKE, D. H. (1962) 'Strength recovery from static and dynamic muscular fatigue'. *Research Quarterly of the American Association for Health, Physical Education and Recreation*, **33**, 349.
12. CLARKE, D. H. (1957). 'Muscular strength endurance relationships'. *Archives of Physical Medicine and Rehabilitation*, **38**, 584.
13. CLARKE, D. H. and PETERSEN, K. H. (1961) 'Contrast of maturational, structural and strength characteristics of athletes and nonathletes 10 to 15 years of age'. *Research Quarterly of the American Association for Health, Physical Education and Recreation*, **32**, 163.
14. CLARKE, D. H. and DEGUTIS, E. W. (1964) 'Relationships between standing broad jump and various maturational, anthropometric and strength tests of 12-year-old boys'. *Research Quarterly of the*

American Association for Health, Physical Education and Recreation, **35**, 258.

15. DAVID, H., HAMLEY, E. J. and THOMAS, V. (1968) 'Analysis of leg muscle action in a repetitive locomotor skill'. *Journal of Physiology*, **197**, 63P.

16. DAWSON, D. M. and ROMANUL, F. C. A. (1964) 'Enzymes in muscle'. *Archives of Neurology*, **11**, 369.

17. DENNY-BROWN, D. and FOLEY, J. M. (1948) 'Myokymia and the benign fasciculation of muscular cramps'. *Transactions of the Association of American Physicians*, **61**, 88.

18. DENNY-BROWN, D. (1953) 'Clinical problems in neuromuscular physiology'. *American Journal of Medicine*, **15**, 368.

19. DE VRIES, H. A. (1961) 'Prevention of muscular distress after exercise'. *Research Quarterly of the American Association for Health, Physical Education and Recreation*, **32**, 177.

20. DE VRIES, H. A. (1961) 'Electromyographic observations of the effects of static stretching upon muscular distress'. *Research Quarterly of the American Association for Health, Physical Education and Recreation*, **32**, 468.

21. DE VRIES, H. A. (1962) 'Evaluation of static stretching procedures for improvement of flexibility'. *Research Quarterly of the American Association for Health, Physical Education and Recreation*, **33**, 222.

22. DUBOWITZ, V. and PEARSE, A. G. (1960) 'Comparative histochemical study of oxidative enzymes and phosphorylase activity in skeletal muscle'. *Histochemie*, **2**, 105.

23. FISCHER, E. and SOLOMAN, S. (1965) 'Physiological responses to heat and cold'. In, *Therapeutic heat*, Ed. S. Licht. Elizabeth Licht: New Haven, Connecticut.

24. FLEISHMAN, E. A. (1964) *The structure and measurement of physical fitness*. Prentice Hall: Englewood Cliffs, New Jersey.

25. GOLLNICK, P. D. and KING, D. W. *Effects of exercise and training on mitochondria of rat skeletal muscle*. Communications.

26. GREEY, S. W. (1955) *A study of the flexibility in five selected joints of adult males, ages 18 to 71*. Ph.D. diss., University of Michigan.

27. GUYTON, A. C. (1969) *Function of the human body*. Saunders: Philadelphia.

28. HAMLEY, E. J. and THOMAS, V. (1968) 'Electromyographic analysis of leg muscle coordination during bicycle pedalling'. *Proceedings of the International Union of Physiological Societies*, **7**, 178.

29. HENRY, F. M. (1954) 'Time velocity equations and oxygen requirements of "all out" and "steady pace" running'. *Research Quarterly of*

the American Association for Health, Physical Education and Recreation, **25**, 164.

30. HENRY, F. M. (1956) 'Motor learning and coordination'. *Proceedings of the College Physical Education Association*, **59**, 68.

31. HENRY, F. M. and WHITLEY, J. D. (1960) 'Relationships between individual differences in strength, speed and mass in arm movement'. *Research Quarterly of the American Association for Health, Physical Education and Recreation*, **31**, 24.

32. HENRY, F. M. *et al.* (1960) 'Factorial structure of speed and static strength in a lateral arm movement'. *Research Quarterly of the American Association for Health, Physical Education and Recreation*, **31**, 440.

33. HENRY, F. M. *et al.* (1962) 'Factorial structure of individual differences in limb speed, reaction, and strength'. *Research Quarterly of the American Association for Health, Physical Education and Recreation*, **33**, 70.

34. HERMANSEN, L. (1969) 'Anaerobic energy release'. *Medicine and Science in Sports*, **1**, 1.

35. HETTINGER, T. and MULLER, E. A. (1953) 'Muskelleistung und Muskeltraining'. *Arbeitsphysiologie*, **15**, 11.

36. HILDEBRAND, M. (1944) 'Motions of the running cheetah and horse'. *Journal of Mammalogy*, **25**, 67.

37. HOLLOSZY, J. O. (1967) 'Effects of exercise on mitochondrial oxygen uptake and respiratory enzyme activity in skeletal muscle'. *Journal of Biological Chemistry*, **242**, 2278.

38. HOOKS, G. (1962) *Application of weight training to athletics.* Prentice Hall: Englewood Cliffs, New Jersey.

39. HOUGH, T. (1902) 'Ergographic studies on muscular soreness'. *American Journal of Physiology*, **7**, 76.

40. HUNT, C. C. (1952) 'The effect of stretch receptors from muscle on the discharge of motoneurons'. *Journal of Physiology*, **117**, 359.

41. IKAI, M. and STEINHAUS, A. H. (1961) 'Some factors modifying the expression of human strength'. *Journal of Applied Physiology*, **16**, 157.

42. INMAN, V. T. *et al.* (1952) 'Relation of human electromyogram to muscular tension'. *EEG and Clinical Neurophysiology*, **4**, 187.

43. KIDD, G. L. and CHARLESWORTH, E. J. (1971; 1972) 'Physiological studies of the effects of endurance training: 1, 2 and 3'. *British Journal of Physical Education*, **2**, 5; **3**, 1.

44. KINGSLEY, D. B. (1952) *Flexibility changes resulting from participation in tumbling.* Master's thesis, University of Oregon.

45. LANDRETH, W. G. (1957) *A comparative study of two methods for improving range of movement.* Master's thesis, University of California.
46. LEIGHTON, J. R. (1964) 'A study of the effect of progressive weight training on flexibility'. *Journal for Physical and Mental Rehabilitation*, **18**, 10.
47. LIBET, B. *et al.* (1955) 'Tendon afferents in autogenetic inhibition'. *Federation Proceedings. Federation of American Societies for Experimental Biology*, **14**, 92.
48. LILIENTHAL, J. L. (1955) 'On muscular cramps'. *Journal of Chronic Disease*, **1**, 100.
49. LOGAN, G. and WALLIS, E. (1960) 'Recent findings in learning and performance'. *Proceedings of the CAHPER Congress, October.*
50. MASSEY, B. H. and CHAUDET, N. L. (1956) 'Effects of systematic, heavy resistance exercise on range of joint movement in young male adults'. *Research Quarterly of the American Association for Health, Physical Education and Recreation*, **27**, 41.
51. MCCOUCH, G. P. *et al.* (1950) 'Inhibition of knee jerk from tendon spindles of crureus'. *Journal of Neurophysiology*, **13**, 343.
52. MERTON, P. A. (1954) 'Voluntary strength and fatigue'. *Journal of Physiology*, **123**, 553.
53. MOUNTCASTLE, V. B. (1961) 'Reflex activity of the spinal cord'. In, *Medical physiology*, Ed. P. Bard, C. V. Mosby: St Louis.
54. NEEDHAM, D. M. (1956) 'Energy production in muscle'. *British Medical Bulletin*, **12**, 194.
55. NORRIS, F. H. *et al.* (1957) 'An electromyographic study of induced and spontaneous muscle cramps'. *EEG and Clinical Neurophysiology*, **9**, 139.
56. O'CONNELL, F. K. (1960) 'The role of weight lifting in athletics'. *Journal of the Association for Physical and Mental Rehabilitation*, **14**, 136.
57. PETREN, T. (1936) 'Der Einfluss des Trainings auf die Haufigkeit der Capillaren in Herz und Skeletmuskulatur'. *Arbeitsphysiologie*, **9**, 376.
58. PUGH, L. G. C. E., CORBETT, J. L. and JOHNSON, R. H. (1967) 'Rectal temperatures, weight losses and sweat rates in marathon running'. *Journal of Applied Physiology*, **23**, 347.
59. RASCH, P. J. (1961) 'Progressive resistance exercise: isotonic and isometric; a review'. *Journal of the Association for Physical and Mental Rehabilitation*, **15**, 2.
60. RATHBONE, J. L. (1954) *Corrective physical education.* W. B. Saunders: Philadelphia.

61. ROBINSON, S. *et al.* (1965) 'Relations between sweating, cutaneous blood flow and body temperature in work'. *Journal of Applied Physiology*, **20**, 575.

62. ROHTER, F. D. and HYMAN, C. (1962) 'Blood flow in arm and finger during muscle contraction, and joint positional changes'. *Journal of Applied Physiology*, **17**, 819.

63. ROMANUL, F. C. A. (1964) 'Enzymes in muscle'. *Archives of Neurology*, **11**, 355.

64. ROYCE, J. (1964) 'Reevaluation of isometric training methods and results, a must'. *Research Quarterly of the American Association for Health, Physical Education and Recreation*, **35**, 125.

65. SALTIN, B. and HERMANSEN, L. (1967) 'Glycogen stores and prolonged severe exercise'. *Symposia on Nutrition*, **V**.

66. SALTIN, B. and GAGGE, A. P. (1968) 'Muscle temperatures during submaximal exercise'. *Federation Proceedings. Federation of American Societies for Experimental Biology*, **27**, 232.

67. SHELDON, W. H. *et al.* (1940) *The varieties of human physique.* Harper: New York.

68. SMITH, L. E. (1961) 'Relationship between explosive leg strength and performance in the vertical jump'. *Research Quarterly of the American Association for Health, Physical Education and Recreation*, **35**, 405.

69. SMITH, L. E. (1961) 'Individual differences in strength, reaction latency, mass and length of limbs, and their relation to maximal speed of movement'. *Research Quarterly of the American Association for Health, Physical Education and Recreation*, **32**, 208.

70. SMITH, L. E. (1964) 'Influence of strength training in pretensed and free arm speed'. *Research Quarterly of the American Association for Health, Physical Education and Recreation*, **35**, 554.

71. STAFFORD, G. T. and KELLY, E. D. (1958) *Preventative and corrective physical education.* Ronald: New York.

72. STAINSBY, W. N. and WELCH, H. G. (1966) 'Lactate metabolism of contracting dog skeletal muscle *in situ*'. *American Journal of Physiology*, **211**, 177.

73. STEINHAUS, A. H. (1933) 'Chronic effects of exercise'. *Physiological Reviews*, **13**, 103.

74. STEINHAUS, A. H. (1963) *Toward an understanding of health and physical education.* William C. Brown Co: Dubuque, Iowa.

75. THOMAS, V. (1971) *The tolerance of extreme physical stress in sportsmen.* Ph.D. thesis, University of Surrey.

76. THOMAS, V. (1971) 'The effects of glucose syrup ingestion on extended locomotor performance'. *British Journal of Sports Medicine*, **5**, 4.

77. THOMAS, V. (1971) 'Some effects of glucose syrup ingestion during vigorous exercises of differing intensities and durations'. *Proceedings of the Nutrition Society*, **31**, 5a.
78. WEBER, S. and KRAUS, H. (1949) 'Passive and active stretching of muscles'. *Physical Therapy Review*, **29**.
79. WHITLEY, J. D. and SMITH, L. E. (1963) 'Velocity curves and static strength–action strength correlations in relation to the mass moved by the arm'. *Research Quarterly of the American Association for Health, Physical Education and Recreation*, **34**, 379.
80. WHITTLE, H. D. (1956) *Effects of elementary school physical education upon some aspects of physical, motor, and personality development of boys twelve years of age*. Ph.D. diss., Eugene, University of Oregon.
81. WRIGHT, S. (1966) *Applied Physiology*. Oxford University Press.

CHAPTER THREE

Circulation

Generally, 'circulation' is used to describe the movement of blood about the body – though there are other substances which also circulate apart from the blood stream. The circulatory system is seen as composed of blood, blood vessels and the heart. The functions of this system in the athlete are to supply oxygen and nutrients to the working tissues, to clear the waste products of combustion, to maintain correct body temperature and to distribute control substances throughout the body.

Blood

Almost all the blood cells are of a type described as red blood cells. Within each cubic millimetre of blood are normally approximately five million red cells, though for the sportsman this figure may be increased by 30 or 40 per cent – a condition termed sports polycythaemia. A deficiency of red blood cells is termed anaemia which, if it is a temporary effect of training, is called sports anaemia. Women have normally somewhat lower red cell counts than men. The volumetric proportion of the red blood cells in the blood is called the haematocrit, which is usually 50 per cent or more in sportsmen.

Red blood cells are formed in bone marrow, the final product being a denucleated cell called an erythrocyte, which

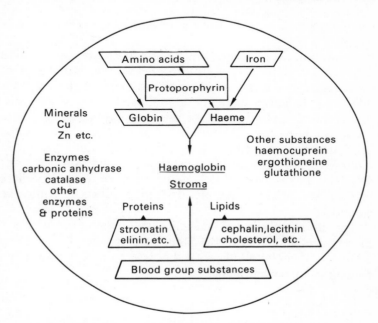

Fig. 3.1 Constituents of the red blood cell (redrawn from Wintrobe, M. M.: *Clinical Hematology*, Lea & Febiger, 1968)

diffuses into the capillaries. Having no nucleus, the cell is incapable of regeneration and has a limited life span of about 120 days. The cell is virtually a membranous bag of haemoglobin (Fig. 3.1).

Haemoglobin content is critically important to the athlete since it is the oxygen-carrying component of the blood. Its active constituent is ferrous iron, which bonds loosely and easily reversibly with oxygen. About 1 milligram of iron per day is excreted. The remainder of the iron released when the blood cell eventually breaks down is retained by the liver or bone marrow to be reused in new blood cells. The production of red blood cells is dependent upon the demand for oxygen in the body, with a time lag of a few days between demand and production. It can be seen that the early phases of a strenuous training can lead to a worsening lag in red cell production which might last for several weeks. This is sports anaemia.

In addition to red blood cells, there are a number of white cells (about 1 to every 500 red cells), which have great importance in the maintenance of health since they combat infectious bacteria. Sometimes confused with white cells, though not actually cells at all, are the blood platelets. These are small particles of a special white cell produced in the bone marrow, and they number about 300,000 per cubic millimetre of blood. Platelets have the property of attaching themselves to the mouth of open wounds, where they rupture and release blood clotting substances into the wound.

The blood cells and platelets are contained in the plasma — the extracellular fluid of the blood. This plasma is similar to other extracellular fluids with the exception that its protein content is somewhat higher.

Oxygen transport

In normal males the average content of haemoglobin in the blood is 15·8 grammes per 100 millilitre, while females have 13·7 g per 100 ml. The average for both sexes is 14·5 g per 100 ml. However, a standard of 14·8 g per 100 ml has been established, and is referred to as 100 per cent haemoglobin. Male and female athletes of international standard have $\bar{x} = 110·7$ per cent and SD = 13·6 per cent.[52] When fully saturated, one gramme of haemoglobin carries 1·34 ml of oxygen. The normal blood volume of an adult is 6 litres, with athletes tending to have somewhat greater volumes.

It can easily be seen that fully oxygenated blood is hypothetically capable of transporting 1·27 litres of oxygen in an average man.

$$\frac{6000 \text{ ml} \times 15\cdot8 \times 1\cdot34 \text{ ml}}{100 \text{ ml}} = 1\cdot27 \text{ litres oxygen}$$

This figure could be increased by 40 per cent or more in male athletes. However, it must be noted that the actual figure is rather less, since normally each 100 ml of arterial blood passed to the tissues carries only about 19 ml of oxygen in combination with haemoglobin (there is also a small amount of 0·3 ml oxygen per 100 ml actually dissolved in the blood). This would give a total carrying capacity of 1·4 litres of oxygen.

The oxygen carried by the blood is not all taken up by tissue function. The differences between the oxygen content of blood leaving the ventricles and of the blood entering the atria is termed the a–v oxygen difference. At any level of oxygen (V_{O_2}), the a–v difference depends on the proportion of cardiac output going to working muscles. If the proportion of blood going to non-working tissues is high then the a–v difference will be small – and vice versa. The a–v difference in athletes is normally in the region of 90 per cent. Therefore, of a total capacity of 1·4 litres of O_2 in the blood, only 1·26 litres would be used.

Carbon dioxide transport

Only approximately 5 per cent of blood carbon dioxide is actually in the dissolved state. The remainder diffuses from the plasma into the red cell, where the bulk of it undergoes a two stage reaction:

(1) carbon dioxide reacts with water to form carbonic acid. This normally slow reaction is accelerated by the enzyme carbonic anhydrase within the red cell.
(2) The acid–base buffers of the cell immediately react with the carbonic acid to convert most of it to bicarbonate ion, thus maintaining the cell acidity near its normal level.

A small part of the carbon dioxide combines directly with the haemoglobin to form carbaminohaemoglobin, but this is a slow reaction and of relatively little importance. It does demonstrate, however, that haemoglobin can act as a simultaneous carrier of oxygen and carbon dioxide.

Nutrients

In sports activity we have seen that energy is provided almost entirely by carbohydrate and fat metabolism. These nutrients are transported by the blood.

Carbohydrate is transported in the form of blood glucose, which is present during normal early morning fasting rest in a concentration of approximately 90 mg per 100 ml. Blood glucose levels fluctuate widely in response to dietary intake and work rate. Glucose is a readily diffusible substance, and there are normally no barriers to its progress through cell membranes. Historically, blood glucose has therefore been taken as an accurate index of intracellular glucose in the working muscles. For example, the blood volume forms approximately one tenth of total body fluid volume, and the blood glucose also forms about a tenth of body fluid glucose.

Fat is also contained in the blood plasma, at a normal level of approximately 700 mg per 100 ml. This fat takes three major forms – mainly fat and fatty acids, as phospholipids, and as cholesterol and cholesterides. Blood fat levels also vary widely with dietary intake and exercise levels.

Lactic acid

During anaerobic work, lactic acid forms in the muscle cells and, being freely diffusible, passes through the cell membrane to enter the blood plasma. The normal resting range of blood lactate is 10–20 mg per 100 ml, but it may rise ten-fold during severe exercise. The blood lactate level is taken to represent the concentration in the muscle cells and the interstitial fluids. There are some doubts that the muscle cell membrane remains permeable to lactate during some forms of

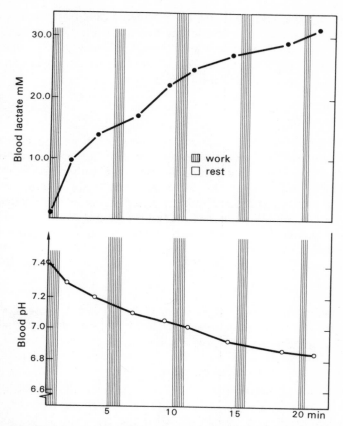

Fig. 3.2 Blood lactate concentration and blood pH before and after each of 5 maximal work periods. The work time varied from 1 min on the first to 35 sec on the fifth period, and the rest periods were 4 min between each work period (from Cerretelli, P.: 'Lactacid oxygen debt in acute and chronic hypoxia', in *Exercise at Altitude*, ed. R. Margaria, Excerpta Medical Foundation, 1967)

strenuous exercise, but this conjecture remains without validation.

We noted earlier that carbon dioxide passing into the blood was buffered and did not cause a significant increase in blood acidity. On the other hand, an increase in blood lactate causes a concomitant increase in blood acidity by increasing the hydrogen ion concentration (Fig. 3.2).

Temperature

Since muscular work releases large amounts of energy as heat at the muscle site, an efficient clearance of the heat has to be achieved by removing it via the blood. Capillaries are immediately adjacent to the working muscle fibres, and heat passes into the blood which then redistributes it throughout the body. More particularly, peripheral blood vessels allow the heat to be lost into the surrounding medium (air or water).

Exchange methods

The passage of energy and chemicals into and out of the blood follows the basic principles discussed in Chapter 1, namely active and passive transport mechanisms.

Mechanics of circulation

The circulation is concerned with the movement of blood around a network of vessels which provide various resistances to its flow. The blood vessels vary from large (at the point where they leave the heart) to microscopically small (in the thin walled capillaries where substance transfer occurs). A diagrammatic representation of the circulatory system is given in Fig. 3.3.

The force necessary to propel blood through the arteries, arterioles and capillaries is provided by the contraction of the heart muscle.

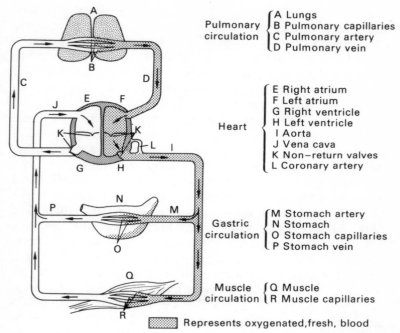

Pulmonary
circulation
{
A Lungs
B Pulmonary capillaries
C Pulmonary artery
D Pulmonary vein
}

Heart
{
E Right atrium
F Left atrium
G Right ventricle
H Left ventricle
I Aorta
J Vena cava
K Non-return valves
L Coronary artery
}

Gastric
circulation
{
M Stomach artery
N Stomach
O Stomach capillaries
P Stomach vein
}

Muscle
circulation
{
Q Muscle
R Muscle capillaries
}

▨ Represents oxygenated, fresh, blood

Fig. 3.3 The circulatory system

The heart

It is common to speak of the heart as a pump, but actually its
four chambers constitute four separate pumps. Each of the
atria acts as a primer pump, ensuring more complete filling of
the ventricles with blood prior to their ejection contraction.
Since little force is required to achieve this priming, the
muscle walls of the atria are relatively thin. Even during atrial
failure, the ventricles are sufficiently powerful to maintain a
large blood supply without priming.

During basal resting conditions, the metabolic demands of
the body tissues require a minimal blood supply. At this level,
the cardiac output is approximately 5 litres of blood per
minute. It is commonly observed that the basal heart rate of
the athlete is considerably lower than that of non-athletes. A

study of several hundred athletes of international standard revealed a mean basal heart rate of 54·12,[52] with certain subgroups achieving much lower rates, e.g. 10 teenage athletes $\bar{x} = 50·5$, $SD = 7·3$; 63 physical education students $\bar{x} = 52·45$, $SD = 5·54$; 20 international rowers $\bar{x} = 45·25$, $SD = 4·71$. These compare with the average value for non-athletes of 72 beats per minute.

Since cardiac output is a product of the number of systolic ejections per minute and the mean volume of blood ejected in each stroke, it can be seen that the basal stroke volumes for the rowers would be approximately $5000/45 = 111$ ml, whereas for a non-athlete it would be $5000/72 = 69$ ml. Basal heart rates for some sportsmen range as low as 32 beats per minute,[53] which would give a basal stroke volume of $5000/32 = 156$ ml. Such calculations are based upon the assumption that there is no significant difference in the basal metabolic demands of the athlete and the non-athlete. In fact, sportsmen have been shown to develop reduced basal cardiac outputs.[28, 36] Radiological determination of the total heart volume in highly trained athletes gives values between 900 and 1400 ml, against volumes of 600–900 ml for non-athletes. This increased volume is due both to a hypertrophy and a lengthening of muscle fibres,[33] which is experienced by all chambers of the heart simultaneously.[40]

The ejection of blood during systole is accomplished by a contraction of the cardiac myofibrils, reducing the intra-cardiac space. The atrial musculature contracts to prime the ventricles, followed shortly by the ventricular musculature which exerts pressure on the ventricular blood. This pressure closes the atrioventricular valve and opens the semilunar valves into the aorta and the pulmonary artery. The resting pressure exerted on the ventricular blood in a study of 147 international class athletes was $\bar{x} = 133·18$, $SD = 13·63$ mmHg.[52] It should be pointed out that this observation is contrary to the findings of other workers that resting systolic pressure is lower in athletes.[32, 39] Immediately prior to ventricular systole (i.e. at the end of diastole), the pressure of the blood remaining within the aorta is low, about 70 mmHg in sportsmen. The ventricular blood flows from the region of high pressure into the low pressure area, where the extremely elastic arterial walls distend to accommodate the extra volume. Upon cessation of ventricular systole, the pressure difference between the ventricles and the arteries is reversed, which closes the aortic valve and prevents blood flowing back into the heart (Fig. 3.4). The cardiac muscle then relaxes,

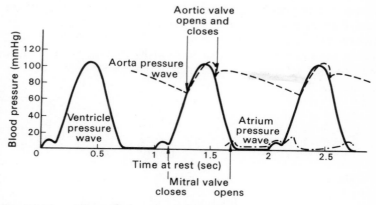

Fig. 3.4 The cardiac cycle in terms of blood pressure

allowing the chambers to return to their larger dimensions and the first influx of blood into atria. The whole operation is termed the cardiac cycle.

Ventricular systole does not normally completely empty the ventricles of blood. At resting levels the cardiac contraction is not a powerful one, and a pool of blood is left within the ventricles. This pool is greater in the trained than the untrained person. During forceful contraction the emptying is more complete in both cases, with the extra blood from the 'cardiac pool' then entering the system – a kind of blood transfusion. It is important to note that the pool also permits a rapid rise in cardiac output without there necessarily having to be a rise in venous return to the heart – at least for the first few beats.

During extremely heavy work, the ventricular systolic pressure in highly trained athletes may rise to more than 250 mmHg. Their reserves of systolic pressure are considerably greater than the non-athlete's!

The difference between systolic and diastolic pressure is termed the pulse pressure. The mean of the two pressures may be termed mean blood pressure. The mean blood pressure can be seen as an expression of the health and age of the circulatory system, within normal limits the lower the better provided the pulse pressure is sufficiently great. Normal figures for healthy young adults would be 120/80 mmHg, giving a mean blood pressure of 100 mmHg with a pulse pressure of 40 mmHg. Studies of athletes show the following pressures:[52]

	$\bar{x}$	SD
systolic pressure	133·18	13·63
diastolic pressure	69·85	9·68
pulse pressure	63·33	13·12

The mean blood pressure of these athletes is:

$$(133·18 + 69·85)/2 = 101·52 \text{ mmHg.}$$

This is not significantly different from normal, and if we take the point in the cardiac cycle where the pressure is normal (i.e. 100 mmHg) we can trace the fluctuations in pressure. The bigger and stronger heart of the athlete causes a higher systolic pressure rise than normal. Because a greater stroke volume is achieved there is a longer recovery period during which the pressure has more time to drop reaching thereby a lower diastolic pressure. The overall effect is an increase in the pulse pressure, which may be taken as an index of cardiac performance. Such cardiac phenomena in athletes are considered to be pathologic by some workers, particularly the great Russian sports scientists Letounov and Motylyanskaya.[31, 32] They argue that hypertension caused through physical over exertion results in little change in diastolic level (from 81 to 90 mmHg) but a great rise in systolic level (from 135 to 177 mmHg). This condition can be seen in 30 per cent

of those young athletes suffering hypertension. The mean
blood pressure in these cases is $(156 + 85)/2 = 120$ mmHg
mercury, which is considerably higher than normal, but not
into the range which might be described as clinically abnormal.

The arteries, arterioles and capillaries

Whereas circulation is commonly referred to in terms of
blood flow (e.g. in litres per minute), it is also important to
consider blood velocity (e.g. in cm per second). If the quantity
of blood flowing through a vessel remains constant, then the
larger the vessel the slower does the blood flow. The main
artery, the aorta, has a cross-sectional area of approximately
2 sq. cm. It then subdivides into smaller vessels (arteries,
arterioles and capillaries), *but at each subdivision the total
cross-sectional area of the system increases* (Fig. 3.4). In fact,
the total cross-sectional area of the arterioles is about 25
times as great as that of the aorta, and of the capillaries, about
750 times. The figures for blood velocity are therefore normally in the order of

aorta	30 cm/sec
arterioles	1·5 cm/sec
capillaries	0·04 cm/sec
venules	0·5 cm/sec
vena cava	8 cm/sec

Since substance and energy transfer occur in the capillaries, it
is important that the blood velocity is sufficiently slow to
enable transfer to take place. Fortunately, during strenuous
performance, the sportsman's working muscle capillaries distend as much as five-fold. Therefore, the great increases in
total blood flow are not directly reflected as increased blood
velocity in the capillaries.

Resistance to flow

The wall of a blood vessel provides a resistance to the passage
of the blood. This resistance, which arises from the friction

between the wall and the blood, has three factors. It is inversely proportional to the length of the vessel and to the viscosity (thickness) of the blood, and proportional to the fourth power of the diameter of the vessel. From these factors, Poiseuille's law was derived:

$$\text{blood flow} \propto \frac{\text{pressure} \times (\text{diameter})^4}{\text{length} \times \text{viscosity}}$$

It can easily be seen that a sportsman's five-fold capillary distension could lead to an increased blood flow of 625-fold *in that capillary.*

Flow shunts

At rest, the circulation of 5 litres per minute in a normal adult is distributed as follows:

	%	ml/min
liver	27	1350
kidneys	22	1100
muscle	15	750
brain	14	700
skin	6	300
bone	5	250
heart	4	200
bronchi	2	100
thyroid	1	50
adrenals	0·5	25
other tissues	3·5	175
	100	5000

As the sportsman exercises, these proportions change, with less vital functions being 'switched off' and more vital functions greatly enhanced. Particularly, there is a peripheral vascular pooling to assist heat flow to the surrounding air, increased splanchnic flow during long duration submaximal work, and increased flow in working muscles (including cardiac muscle which shows a ten-fold increase). There is some evidence that even with a gross increase in working muscle blood flow, the *proportion* of blood flow to the muscle may decrease while the splanchnic proportion increases.[17, 37] This phenomenon is compatible with a lower level of muscular work and higher level of constant energy supply from the liver − as seen in the distance runner. On the other hand, in some extremely strenuous short duration activities, local muscle blood flow may increase fifteen-fold, with total muscle flow representing 75 per cent of the circulation.[18]

The location of blood at any given moment demonstrates that at rest only a small proportion of the blood is in a situation where substance and energy transfer can take place.

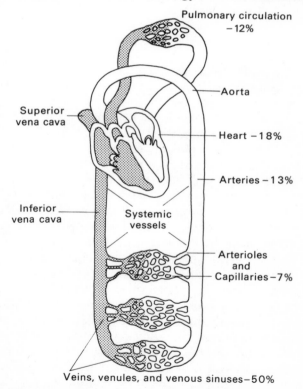

Fig. 3.5 Distribution of blood in the different parts of the circulatory system

At rest, the capillaries contain only a few per cent of the blood (Fig. 3.5).

The control of the blood flow shunts is achieved through the arterioles, which account for one half of the total flow resistance in the systemic circulation. Changes in arteriole diameter have a greater effect on blood flow in a given location than any other vessel diameter changes. The precise method by which this control is achieved has not yet been determined, but one major theory is that the arteriolar muscular wall needs oxygen to maintain its tonic constriction of the arteriole. When the oxygen supply is taken up by surrounding muscular tissue, the arteriole muscle relaxes thus dilating the arteriole itself.

Veins and venules

Blood escapes from the capillary bed under a relatively low pressure, and with a virtual cessation of the pulsar propulsion from the heart. When standing, an athlete's venous system might very well be 120 cm long. This means that if there were no breaks in that column, there would be a hydrostatic pressure of 120 cm blood, plus the various fluid resistances, plus the pressure within the right atrium, to be overcome before blood could return to the heart. In some cases this can total 100 mmHg, a force which the remaining pulse pressure is absolutely unable to overcome. Fortunately, the veins are interrupted at intervals by valves which support the column of blood above them as far as the next valve. If one of these valves fails, the greater pressure of the longer column of blood causes distension of the veins and a pooling in the lower circulation — commonly called varicose veins.

In the healthy vein the effect of the valves is that blood can only flow towards the heart, and the effect of working muscles is to squeeze the veins, thus causing a rise in pressure which forces the blood towards an area of lower pressure further up the system. This system is called the muscle pump (Fig. 3.6).

The effects of pressures within the circulatory system are critical. Most of the cardiovascular capacity lies below the

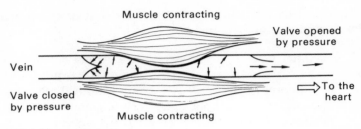

Fig. 3.6 The muscle pump

heart when an athlete is in an erect position. Hydrostatic pressures then assist arterial circulation (i.e. the function of the heart), and hinder venous pressures (i.e. the function of the muscle pump). In activities where the lower leg is active, this will be sufficient to ensure venuous return, and an erect position will aid cardiac function. This is particularly true after strenuous cardiac exercise when recovery should be made while walking or jogging. On the other hand, recovery from exhausting local muscular effort will be better if the limb involved is elevated to assist venuous return.

Oxygen uptake

The combination of several factors forms a physiological parameter of paramount importance in sports performance. This is maximum oxygen uptake (V_{O_2}max)

$$\dot{V}_{O_2} = \text{cardiac output} \times \text{a–v difference}$$
where   cardiac output = stroke volume × heart rate
and   a–v difference = ml O_2 extracted per ml blood

At maximum work levels, the large trained heart of a sportsman can reach outputs of 40 l/minute, with stroke volumes of 200 ml and heart rates of 200/min. The maximal a–v difference of trained athletes is approximately 18 ml per 100 ml. We therefore have

maximal V_{O_2} = 200 × 200 × $\frac{18}{100}$ ml per minute
= 7·2 litres, which is just a little greater than that recorded on superbly conditioned German oarsmen.[1]

Figures from Astrand[6] and Saltin[43] for student sportsmen after several years of training are

maximal V_{O_2}	4·93 l/min
	64 ml/kg/min
a–v difference	17·1 ml/100 ml
maximal cardiac output	28·9 l/min
maximum heart rate	186 beats/min
maximum stroke volume	155 ml

Earlier we saw that aerobic muscular function is that which proceeds in the presence of oxygen (pp. 40–1). The limit of oxygen uptake by the body tissues therefore constitutes a limit to aerobic muscular function. V_{O_2} is generally accepted as being one of the most important indices of physical fitness, being viewed not only as an absolute measure (valuable in events where total work done is the criterion) but also as a relative measure (of importance when considering events where body weight is a relative resistance). The latter measure can be expressed as oxygen uptake per unit body weight per minute (ml/kg/min), with outstanding athletes recording as high as 85 ml/kg/min.[44]

The energy released when a litre of oxygen 'burns' each of the three basic nutrients amounts to

carbohydrates	5·05 calories
fats	4·70 calories
proteins	4·60 calories

An average figure of 4·825 calories is used to represent the combustion of nutrients with one litre of oxygen. In this case the maximal aerobic function of a superathlete will be

$$7·2 \times 4·825 = 34·74 \text{ calories per minute}$$

When one considers that the energy requirement for very severe exercise in a normal male is 10 calories per minute, the term 'superathlete' does not appear extreme.

Carbon dioxide release

Parallel with the oxygen uptake system there is another which deals with the production and dispersal of carbon dioxide. Its dimensions are similar, since it is essentially concerned with venuous return and carbon dioxide levels, thus

$V\text{CO}_2$ = cardiac output (pulmonary circulation)
$\times$ a–v difference (CO_2)

The use of the pulmonary circulation is of course arbitrary, since cardiac output is the same from either ventricle, and is also equal to venuous return to either atrium – apart from transient differences due to time lags in the control mechanisms of the heart. However, it reflects the fact that arterial levels of carbon dioxide are high and venous levels low in the pulmonary circulation. We shall see later that it is to the blood carbon dioxide levels that many of the sportsman's control systems respond.

Though similar in dimensions, the time course of blood carbon dioxide levels is not always parallel with oxygen levels. The lactic acid which accumulates in the plasma during strenuous exercise is buffered by bicarbonate, resulting in the liberation of large amounts of carbon dioxide and water without any equivalent utilisation of oxygen. This process is superimposed on the normal oxygen usage and carbon dioxide formation during muscle work.

Respiratory quotient

The relation between oxygen uptake and carbon dioxide production is termed the respiratory quotient (RQ)

$$RQ = \text{CO}_2 \text{ production}/\text{O}_2 \text{ production}$$

At rest the RQ is generally about $0 \cdot 8$, increasing to about $0 \cdot 9$ in moderate exercise. In strenuous exercise, the excess carbon dioxide production causes the RQ to rise above unity, and is some index of the degree of exertion. RQ can rise as high as $2 \cdot 0$ during extreme exertion.

During rest following violent exercise, muscle lactate is disposed of by reoxidation to pyruvate and dissimilation to carbon dioxide and water (plus a small amount reconverted to glycogen). The carbon dioxide thus formed enters the blood and is retained there to a great extent to reform the bicarbonate which was used during exercise, rather than being immediately expelled through the lungs. The RQ therefore (which is usually measured by inspired and expired air mixtures) attains much lower values during the recovery period.

Blood lactate

The resting level of lactic acid in the blood lies between 10 and 20 mg/100 ml. Having established that base level, a rational explanation of blood lactate levels is not yet forthcoming. A great deal of conflicting evidence is available, from which certain fundamental lactate reactions can be established. Normally muscle cell membranes are permeable to lactate, and the production of lactate by moderate or heavy muscle work is demonstrated by a rise in blood lactate. This phenomenon is associated with a demand for oxygen in excess of the capability of the body to supply it. However, there are other causes of lactate formation and indeed a system for lactate reutilisation in the muscle cell itself, which complicate the matter.

During extremely strenuous competition an athlete's blood lactate level may exceed 200 mg/100 ml, and at this level the total body lactate accumulation is approximately 90 g. During rest the blood lactate slowly returns to normal, sometimes needing several hours to complete the process.

If long duration submaximal activity precedes the high intensity work, there is no great change from normal in the final blood lactate level. There is some evidence that this is due to an uptake of lactate by the resting and working muscles,[50] though other research has demonstrated that short duration maximal effort following prolonged severe exercise produces low blood lactate levels which are not caused by muscular lactate usage.[17] The ability to produce (or tolerate) a high blood lactate level increases with endurance training, but no studies have succeeded in demonstrating that blood lactate level (or an inability to depress that level) is a limiting factor in sports performance.

Blood glucose

The normal level of blood glucose after (say) a night's sleep and before breakfast is 90 mg/100 ml. Blood glucose levels alter quickly after ingestion of carbohydrate which becomes available in the peripheral circulation within 20 minutes. Values as high as 250 mg/100 ml are commonly observed in sportsmen, though in normal subjects such a level would indicate a clinical condition.[54] Glucose is readily diffusable throughout body tissues and, while only 5 g may be in the blood (100 mg/100 ml × 5 litres) at a given time, the total content of the body fluids may be 50 g. The comparatively large size of the glucose pool enables it to act as a buffer during competition, minimising variations in blood glucose. For example, irrespective of the amount of carbohydrate taken in, the maximum intestinal sugar absorption rate is approximately 2 g/min. Nearly 4 calories of energy are released by the oxidation of 1 g of glucose. Therefore, continuous ingestion of glucose can only supply 8 calories per minute to the sportsman, and in most competitive situations he is required to draw on his glucose pool. As exhaustion proceeds, the level of blood glucose drops and true exhaustion would be reached in the event of an absolute disappearance of blood glucose. It is doubtful that this level is ever reached in sport though studies have shown blood glucose levels lower than 50 mg/100 ml in exhausted men.[8]

Since it has been established that muscle glycogen can be virtually depleted at exhaustion,[8, 9] and especially that at high effort (50–80 per cent of Vo_2max) work time is closely correlated to initial glycogen content of working muscle, it appears unlikely that the blood glucose levels constitute a limiting factor in sport performance.

Blood lipids (fats)

The blood normally contains fats in the following proportions

neutral fat and fatty acids	200–450 mg/100 ml
phospholipids	150–250 mg/100 ml
cholesterol and cholesterides	150–250 mg/100 ml

An average figure of 500 mg/100 ml of blood gives a total blood lipid content of 25 gm, compared with a total body store of perhaps 1 kg. Since combustion of fat produces 9·4 Cal per gram, the fat store has enough potential energy to keep a sportsman going for some weeks. This fat store can break down to free fatty acids and be supplied by the blood to working tissues. Some studies indicate fat as a preferred energy source during submaximal exercise such as long distance running.[54, 55] In such cases the level of blood fats may rise to 30 mg/100 ml, reflecting the release both of fats from adipose tissue and of breakdown fats by the liver. These fats are used to spare the available glucose, rather than to form more glucose since the carbohydrate to fat transformation is largely not reversible. Though the ability of the blood to carry fat is limited by comparison with its capacity for carbohydrate, the rapid turnover of fat and its greater energy yield (double that of glucose) ensure that it can meet the demands of submaximally working muscles.

Fluctuations in peripheral circulatory fat levels are less predictable than levels of glucose, and close relationships between these and various types and levels of sporting performance have not been established.

Blood amino acids and protein

The total concentration of all 23 amino acids in the blood amounts to only about 30 mg/100 ml, the concentration being buffered by the liver. The derivation of energy from amino acids is initiated in the liver where deamination takes place. The waste product of this process is eventually converted with carbon dioxide into urea, the presence of which in the blood, but more particularly in the urine, is an index of the degree of long-term physical stress being experienced by a sportsman. Protein energy does not make a significant contribution to sports function.

Circulatory adaptation

In considering the way in which the circulation adapts to changes in the demands imposed on the sportsman in training and competition, it is necessary to have some reference level. The most stable reference level is basal metabolic rate, that is, when the sportsman is functioning virtually as a vegetable – usually during deep sleep which is achieved after five or six hours and when the brain is not experiencing the periodic excitations which are characterised by rapid eye movements,[2] and at least 12 hours after a meal. At this time, the metabolism of an average adult amounts to 1 Cal per kg per hour, though it is more closely related to body surface area than to height or weight. There may be considerable differences of basal metabolism in people of greatly differing ages, between the sexes and in different states of health. However, in individuals similar in these respects, the basal metabolism commonly varies by less than 10 per cent. An athlete weighing 70 kg will therefore be likely to have a basal metabolic rate of 70 kg × 1 Cal/hr = 70 Cal/hr or $1 \cdot 17$ Cal/min. To produce each calorie requires the consumption of approximately 200 ml O_2, which gives a basal oxygen uptake of 234 ml O_2/min. With a resting a–v oxygen difference of 5 ml/100 ml, basal cardiac output is then $4 \cdot 680$ l/min. With a basal heart rate of 35/min, stroke volume could then be 128 ml.

If we then examine the same athlete at a high rate of aerobic metabolic performance, we find increases in the various parameters as tabulated.

	Body weight	Metabolic rate	Oxygen uptake	a–v O$_2$ difference	Cardiac output	Stroke volume	Heart rate
units	kg	kcal/min	ml/min	ml/100 ml	ml/min	ml	beats/min
rest	70	1·17	234	5	4·680	128	35
work	70	25·50	5100	17	30·000	180	167
increase	—	21·8x	21·8x	3·4x	6·4x	1·4x	4·8x

These figures are all well within the maximum and the minimum reported from studies with sportsmen. Examination of each parameter gives some indication of the potential for metabolic rate increase during competition.

Oxygen uptake

The curve of increasing oxygen uptake with increasing work done by well motivated athletes reaches a plateau which represents Vo$_2$max for that individual (Fig. 3.7). Figures as high as 7 l/min have been recorded,[1] representing a 28-fold increase in function over basal level. This curve is linear while work is aerobic, but at higher levels of performance the

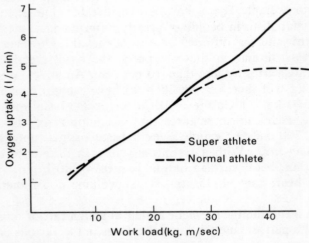

Fig. 3.7 Oxygen uptake with increasing work

work becomes progressively more anaerobic, with all increase beyond V_{O_2}max being due to an increase in anaerobic work.

When work is at a constant level, oxygen uptake increases more sharply to a level which is sufficient to cope with body oxygen needs (Fig. 3.8). However, it is important to be aware that the circulatory response to increases in work load is not immediate. During the time when cardiac output lags behind

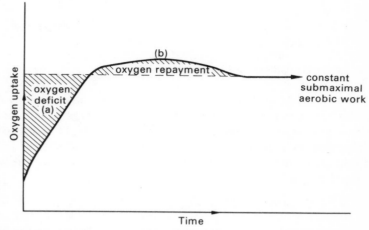

Fig. 3.8 Oxygen uptake at the beginning of constant submaximal aerobic work

what is necessary for a given work load, an oxygen deficit is being incurred. If that load is submaximal then for some time the oxygen supply needs also to clear the oxygen deficit. In Fig. 3.9 this deficit clearance is shown to be equal in magnitude to the deficit accumulation, and the V_{O_2} returns to a steady state which is sufficient to cope with the submaximal metabolic demands. This function represents the circulatory contribution to the athletic phenomenon known as second wind. The repayment of the oxygen deficit is dependent upon the degree to which an athlete can increase his V_{O_2} above the metabolic steady state level. If that level is very close to, or above, the athlete's V_{O_2}max *then he cannot repay the deficit.* The implications for middle distance performers are obvious

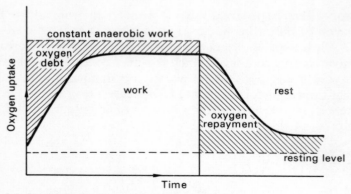

Fig. 3.9 Oxygen uptake during constant anaerobic work

and vital to the athlete's success (Fig. 3.9). In the case shown, a 400 m sprint, the total requirement for oxygen over and above that actually supplied during work is termed the oxygen debt, and this is repaid during the recovery period, which might last minutes or hours. These examples are necessarily simplified, since

(i) *work* never ceases abruptly, since at high levels of effort the energy cost of ventilation is a large part of the total work load, and increased ventilation continues after exercise;

(ii) competitive energy output is rarely constant over more than fractions of a minute – the energy requirements fluctuate;

(iii) during anaerobic work, 1 g of glucose forms 2 g of lactic acid, releasing 0·6 Calories corresponding to the consumption of 120 ml of oxygen. During recovery approximately twice as much oxygen is required to remove the lactate, therefore the actual oxygen repaid is *twice* the oxygen debt.[3, 13]

Oxygen uptake, therefore constitutes a limiting factor in aerobic (submaximal) activities. The effects of competition at work loads in excess of Vo_2max are critical, most particularly the opportunities of recovery from anaerobia during the event and the disadvantages of the extra oxygen demands incurred for repayment of the oxygen debt.

Arterio–venous oxygen difference

Since a–v oxygen difference is a constituent of Vo_2, it follows a substantially similar curve (Fig. 3.10). Values as high as

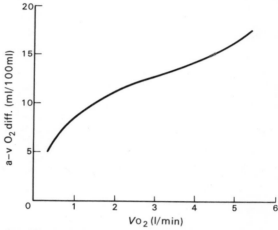

Fig. 3.10 The relationship between a–v oxygen difference and Vo_2

18 ml/100 ml have been recorded, i.e. 90 per cent of the 20 ml/100 ml normally found in arterial blood. Even when blood shunting to working muscles accounts for 80–90 per cent of cardiac output, and that blood is almost drained of oxygen, there is sufficient flow to the skin and other areas of low oxygen uptake to ensure that *mixed* venous blood does not reach greater than 90 per cent dissociation of oxygen. Low levels of a–v oxygen difference do not appear to constitute a limiting factor to sports performance, except in anaemia.[49]

Cardiac output

Again, cardiac output is a constituent of the Vo_2 equation and follows a substantially similar curve (Fig. 3.11). The relation

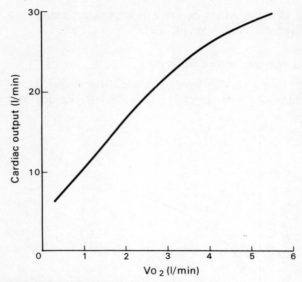

Fig. 3.11 The relationship between cardiac output and V_{O_2}

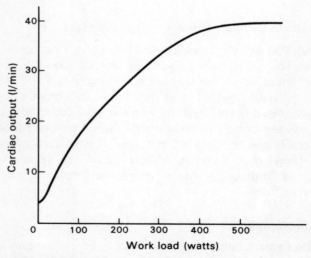

Fig. 3.12 Cardiac output during regularly increasing work

between cardiac output and V_{O_2} is linear up to about 70 per cent of V_{O_2}max, the regression equation for cardiac output being, cardiac output $= 6·01\ V_{O_2} + 3·07$, demonstrating that output increases 6 litres to achieve each 1 litre increase in oxygen uptake. Over the upper 30 per cent of the V_{O_2} curve, the contribution of a–v oxygen difference accelerates to a small degree.

The cardiac output in relation to regularly increasing work load is curvilinear and apparently asymptotic (Fig. 3.12).

The distribution of the cardiac output towards the upper limits of sporting performance is altered by a change in the shunting mechanisms. Particularly, during prolonged work the cooling shunt is maintained to the body surface but in the last resort this mechanism is sacrificed in favour of muscular regions, or in some cases (e.g. during heavy nutrient usage) also in favour of splanchnic flow.

Maximum cardiac output responds to training, improvements of 4·4, 8·0 and 16·4 per cent being noted in longitudinal studies of the training of young men of sedentary occupation.[16, 41, 45] Maximum values of 40 l/min have been recorded in superathletes.[13] Since oxygen uptake constitutes a limiting factor to sports performance, and a–v oxygen difference does not, cardiac output must be a limiting factor.

Stroke volume

This is the first of the two determinants of cardiac output. During brief periods of exercise there is a fine balance between resistance and capacitance blood vessels; this balance holds constant the filling pressure of the right heart. Stroke volume is then maintained in spite of increases in heart rate.

During prolonged work at constant submaximal loads, the equation, $V_{O_2} = $ heart rate $\times$ stroke volume $\times$ a–v oxygen difference, is held with minor changes in the heart rate and stroke volume compensating each other. Stroke volume is increased by perhaps 40 per cent from basal to cater for the constant work load, and then varies very little.

Under the stress of very heavy prolonged competition, the

circulatory shunt to the periphery results in a fall in cardiac filling pressure, central blood volume and *thus in stroke volume*.

In earlier days there was a theory that at very high heart rates the heart had insufficient refilling time and thus suffered a reduced stroke volume. While this is probably true at pathologically high heart rates and during cardiac fibrillation, the maintenance of stroke volumes and cardiac output at heart rates in excess of 200/min has been demonstrated by several workers, particularly in Russian Institutes by Letounov, Rosenblat and Solonin.

The general picture of stroke volume is, then, an initial rise in response to exercise to values which may exceed 200 ml in highly trained sportsmen. There is then a maintenance of stroke volume with only minor changes during strenuous competition of various types, irrespective of the cardiac output and heart rate (Fig. 3.13). In this case, maximum stroke volume is a factor which can be developed by training and which has a limiting function in aerobic performance.

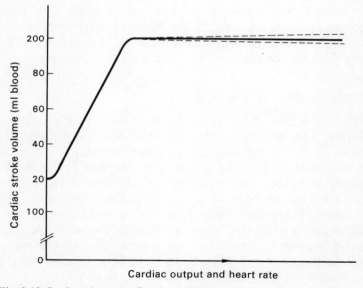

Fig. 3.13 Stroke volume as a function of heart rate

Heart rate

Studies of the response of heart-rate to exercise have always been bedevilled by the sensitivity of heart-rate control mechanisms to conditions other than exercise levels. In particular, psychological, thermal, hormonal, barometric and clinical influences may cause increases in heart rate which exceed those caused by heavy exercise. Experimentation has required the standardisation of non-exercise conditions to a very fine level, and such requirements have not always been met.

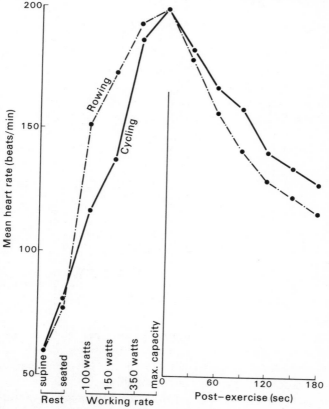

Fig. 3.14 Mean heart rates of 16 international standard oarsmen at various work loads to exhaustion

Measurements of heart rate by palpation of some peripheral artery (radial or carotid) or by direct or telemetered electrocardiography have the benefits of extreme accuracy and ease of monitoring. They constitute the most widespread monitoring methods used in sports science.

In standardised conditions the heart-rate response of sportsmen to constantly increasing work load is linear over most of its range (Fig. 3.14). Here we see the linearity of the

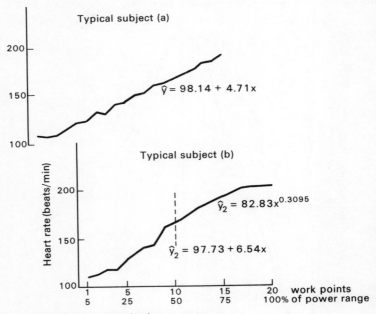

Fig. 3.15 Typical exhaustion heart rate curves

relationship up to approximately 90 per cent of the total increase in heart rate, and then a curvilinear deceleration of heart-rate increase up to exhaustion. In many events the initial acceleration phase is accomplished in 10–15 seconds, representing the start of an 800 m track race for example. In these exercise tests, on international oarsmen, the subjects were well motivated, accustomed to the activity and permitted to stop working only when physiological collapse was imminent. An examination of typical heart-rate curves at exhaustion has revealed that sportsmen can be divided into those whose curves approach an asymptote and those whose curves do not (Fig. 3.15).[11]

The fact that some sportsmen can continue to elevate their heart rate during exhaustion has been well demonstrated by many authors.[5, 13, 23, 42] The levels usually quoted for asymptotes of heart rate are so far below levels observed in competing sportsmen that it is surprising that they should be considered as true maxima. Subjects whose curves do reach apparent maxima are likely to be performing at less than their true exhaustion level – perhaps through psychological inhibition, mechanical inefficiency or some other reason.

Heart rate seems in fact to be a reflection of the total demand on the sportsman, perhaps the best definition being the level of stress he is experiencing. If the stress continues to rise then so will the heart rate whether that stress is physical, physiological or psychological. However, the Vo_2 equation demonstrates that if heart rate continues to increase and Vo_2max remains constant, then either a–v oxygen difference or cardiac stroke volume must diminish. During psychological stimulus it is probable that stroke volumes do not increase at all, and during extreme exhaustion it is also possible that stroke volume decreases somewhat, and that a–v oxygen difference diminishes perhaps due to the greater velocity of blood through the tissues. Conclusive evidence on these phenomena is not yet available.

A study of two sportsmen, which involved manipulating the end work load of an exhausting exercise test so that they could continue to make maximum effort (under intense motivation) even though their actual work output was decreasing, gave the data shown in Table 3.1.[52]

Using such methods it was possible not only to increase the absolute level of maximum heart rate, but also to achieve a 'last gasp' increase from a subject who had hung on grimly to an extremely high plateau for nearly two minutes.

It appears, therefore, that heart rate does not constitute a

TABLE 3.1   *Terminal and recovery heart rates of two subjects, work load being manipulated*

Subject	Minutes	AGP HR	AY HR
	6½		201
	6		202
	5½		202
	5		204
pre-end exercise	4½	201	206
	4	203	207
	3½	203	209
	3	204	211
	2½	205	212
	2	207	215
	1½	208	215
	1	213	215
	½	213	215
	end	215	218
	½	198	196
recovery	1	177	165
	1½	170	147
	2	157	135
age		19	21
maximum work rate		41 kg.m per sec	44 kg.m per sec

limiting factor in aerobic exercise, and does not constitute a limiting factor *per se* in anaerobic exercise.

From p. 88 we saw that an increase of 2000 per cent in oxygen uptake was achieved by increases of 240 per cent in a–v oxygen difference, 540 per cent in cardiac output, 40 per cent in stroke volume and 380 per cent in heart rate. Looking at it in another way

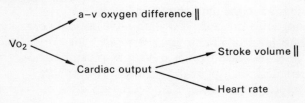

where $\parallel$ represents a limit imposed by the specific physical state of training the sportsman has achieved. The limits to aerobic function at any given time are therefore a–v oxygen difference and stroke volume. These however do not exist as direct limits of anaerobic function, which is a local muscular and psychologically bound function. The heart rate itself does not constitute a limit to performance. It does, however, reflect (a) the level of aerobic function and (b) the degree of total stress being experienced by the sportsman.

Aerobic function

Since heart rate is linearly related to work rate over most of the range from standing motionless erect to V_{O_2}max in the erect position, an individual's heart-rate reaction to submaximal work loads can be extrapolated to his maximal aerobic limit. Unless each individual has established his V_{O_2}max and the heart rate accompanying it, such extrapolation methods depend upon an assumption of normality of these two factors. Most sportsmen are not normal in the physiological sense, being 'super-normal' in many of their performance parameters. Such tests as the Astrand–Rhyming nomogram [5] and others [4, 22, 29, 34, 35, 48, 61] are not intended as predictive tools in sports science but mainly as mass survey techniques for predicting V_{O_2}max. However, heart-rate reaction to a standard submaximal work load can be used to differentiate levels of sporting fitness without necessarily involving predictions of V_{O_2}max, with low validity on a between-subjects basis but with greater validity on a test–retest basis for an individual sportsman. Tests of outstanding professional sportsmen have revealed a fall in heart rate in response to a standard workload test designed by Astrand,[5] i.e. treadmill run at 1 per cent grade at 10 km per hour – over a one month training programme. With 32 subjects the mean heart rate fell from

to $\qquad$ $\bar{x} = 158, SD = 9$

$\bar{x} = 132 \qquad SD = 7.$ [56]

In these cases, such a large fall in heart rate must be accounted for by an increase in stroke volume, and when taken to its lower limit the heart rate of the fitter sportsman is still lower than the less fit in respect of an increased stroke volume. Differences in basal heart rates between different types of sportsmen reflect the physiological demands of their activities.[57]

average man	72	sprinter	58
cricketer	70	footballer	55
fencer	68	oarsman	50
weightlifter	65	swimmer	40
volleyballer	60	runner (2–6 miles)	35

Basal heart rates tend to fall as a result of strenuous training and a drop in an individual sportsman's heart rate is one reflection of increasing fitness. Studies of three groups of sportsmen exposed to varying durations of strenuous training revealed falls in basal heart rate (see Table 3.2).[52]

Stress tolerance

At extreme levels of performance the sportsman has to endure a high level of anaerobiosis. The preceding discussions have demonstrated that the parameters with limits cannot be used to monitor anaerobic performance. On the other hand, heart rate does increase in relation to stress and workers in various countries have examined the use of heart-rate increase over basal level as an index of an increase in tolerance of exercise stress.[21, 27, 42, 60] My own study of this concept[52] has indicated that an index based upon an increase in heart rate over basal is valid in assessing the extent to which an athlete can precipitate and tolerate extreme stress. For convenience this index has been formulated into a cardiac assessment factor (CAF)[58]

$$CAF = \frac{\text{maximum achievable heart rate}}{\text{basal heart rate}} \times 10$$

The three groups mentioned earlier also demonstrated changes in their maximum heart rates, and changes in their CAF.

TABLE 3.2 *Changes in basal and maximum heart rate and in CAF resulting from strenuous training*

		Athletes	PE students	Oarsmen
n		10	65	20
Age, x̄		14·9	19·9	24·5
Age, SD		1·8	1·1	2·3
Length of training		13 months	10 months	3 months
HR_{min}	Test	55·2	58·8	47·7
	Retest	50·5	52·5	45·3
HR_{max}	Test	195·1	190·6	186·6
	Retest	183·1	186·9	193·8
CAF	Test	35·53	32·3	39·2
	Retest	36·9	35·6	42·8

Both the young athletes and the physical education students experienced reduced maximum heart rates, being probably a reflection of maturation processes and a lack of high stress training. On the other hand the international standard oarsmen had very great amounts of high stress training, and experienced a considerable rise in maximum heart rate. However, the overall increase in CAF recorded by all three groups is a reflection of training effects, and the high specificity of CAF in recording effects of high stress tolerance training is clearly demonstrated.

Recovery from exercise

Sports performances may be classified into various types of effort (Fig. 3.16). In some of these categories circulatory recovery is critical (E, F and middle distance), in others it is

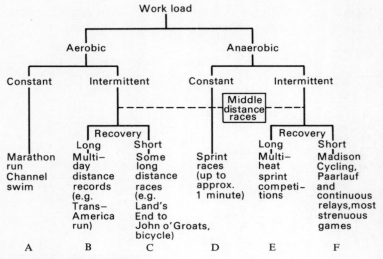

Fig. 3.16 Classes of effort in sport

of lesser importance (A, B, C, D). Circulatory recovery itself may be subdivided into short and long duration, and also the special case of recovery lag.

Short duration   In almost all cases the recovery of the circulation from strenuous exercise is characterised by a rapid fall in heart rate (Fig. 3.17).

We have seen that the compliance of the circulation to heavy exercise lies mainly in the heart rate, rather than a–v oxygen difference and stroke volume. The initial very steep drop in the heart-rate curve is a reflection of this compliance, and when the heart rate has returned to 'medium range' all three circulatory parameters continue the slower task of metabolic recovery. The drop is so steep as to cause doubts that it gives a 'second by second' indication of falling metabolic demand; certainly other parameters do not recover so quickly (lactate, ventilation, temperature, etc.). There is no good evidence that a heart-rate recovery from 195 to 160 within a minute of end of exercise is an indication of a metabolic recovery of 100 (195–160)/195 = 18 per cent.

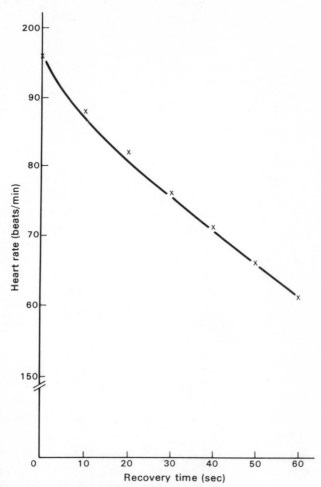

Fig. 3.17 Heart rate recovery from strenuous exercise

However, groups of international class sportsmen from different activities do record different recovery rates over the first
minute of recovery from maximal exhaustive exercise (Table
3.3).[56]

It is noticeable that sportsmen whose approach to exhaustion has been long and gradual, indicating a very great drain

TABLE 3.3   *Heart rate recovery rates*

Category of sport	% maximum heart rate recovered	
	30 sec rest	60 sec rest
Games player	10·1	18·0
Long distance	9·3	16·7
Middle distance	11·2	20·9
Explosive *	5·2	11·7

* Explosive competitors' heart rates sometimes continue to rise *after* finishing their performance.

on body fuel reserves, may experience a short-duration heart-rate recovery of 20 per cent and still be unable to undertake further severe exercise; while those whose exhaustion has led to similar high heart rates but over a short and extremely severe exercise period *can* begin to work again after 20 per cent heart-rate recovery.

For competitors whose short-duration recovery is very important (Fig. 3.15) the heart rate at certain time intervals after the end of exhausting exercise may be used as a criterion of recovery fitness. Indeed, probably the most widely used test of fitness, the Harvard Step Test,[12] is based upon this factor. Using heart-rate recovery measured in absolute values after a set work load which is demanding for some but not for others, the recovery rates being established at $1–1\frac{1}{2}$, $2–2\frac{1}{2}$, $3–3\frac{1}{2}$ minutes after exercise, it has been found that different types of sportsman record different indices, e.g.

pentathlon	154	volleyball	112
basketball	128	judo	111
rowing	123	hockey	106
swimming	122	athletics	105
cycling	121	fencing	96
football	117	weightlifting	95
canoeing	115	gymnastics	93
boxing	115	yachting	92
wrestling	114	equestrianism	86
water polo	112	shooting	83

In these cases there is an apparent difference in Harvard Index between sports relative to the total circulatory demands of the activities, but not a difference relative to the short-duration recovery characteristics of the sports. There are two reasons for this: firstly, the test takes no account of the actual exercise capacity of each subject and therefore is directly related to the absolute level of the heart-rate response to exercise, which itself is a function of efficiency and capacity of the heart; secondly, the heart rates are not expressed in terms of recovery percentage. The test is therefore a more valid test of circulatory efficiency during submaximal exercise than of short-term recovery from maximal exercise.

In general, there is not a widely validated test of short-term circulatory recovery in sportsmen. It remains for each coach to devise his own test, with his own norms, for the sportsmen with whom he deals.

An examination of the short-term heart-rate recovery characteristics following maximal exercise does demonstrate a fairly typical pattern which allows the maximum exercise heart rate to be extrapolated with a high degree of accuracy (Table 3.4).[58]

TABLE 3.4   *Standard error in calculating maximum exercise heart rate by extrapolation from post-exercise rate*

Time elapsed since end of exercise sec	Standard error of calculation beats/min
5	2·839
10	3·507
15	4·265
20	4·642
25	5·187
30	5·854
35	6·550
40	6·770
45	7·202
50	7·590
55	7·913
60	8·281

The sooner heart rate can be measured during the recovery curve, the more accurate is the extrapolation. Indeed, with practice coaches can be trained to measure heart rates by palpation within five seconds of the end of exercise. The maximum heart rate is then given by a formula obtained from a single regression between maximum exercise heart rate and recovery heart rate five seconds post exercise:

$$HR_{max} = 0.98059 \; HR_{pe5sec} + 5.94815$$

The estimate obtained in this way has a standard error of 2.839 beats per minute, which compares with 3.507 at ten seconds post exercise, 4.642 at twenty seconds, 5.854 at thirty and 8.281 at sixty seconds. Similar regression between the end exercise heart rate and 5 seconds post exercise heart rate gives a standard error of 2.485. Though the end exercise heart rate is not always the *maximum* exercise heart rate, the difference is so slight in a well-structured test as to lead to a difference in HR_{max} estimation error of only 0.354 beats.

Long duration   Long duration circulatory recovery can be defined as that part of the recovery curve which is concerned with metabolic recovery. Essentially it begins from the moment exercise ceases, modified by the short-term curve described previously. The accumulation of oxygen debt and of acid exercise products has also been described previously, and the clearance of these conditions is accomplished by an increased cardiac output. Some sportsmen develop the ability to tolerate very high levels of fatigue, which may be measured by lactate levels and oxygen debt levels.[24] At the same absolute rate of recovery, it would be expected that the sportsmen fitter in respect of fatigue tolerance would require longer to recover to resting levels of circulatory function. Since this recovery takes a long time, and is complicated by post-exercise diet, activity levels, etc. it is difficult to discriminate levels of long-term recovery fitness between sportsmen and to correlate these levels with comparative performances. Post-exercise recovery in terms of blood glucose levels and heart rate has been demonstrated to improve significantly with specific dietary intake of glucose syrup before and during exercise.[55]

Since a high level of cardiac output is dependent on venous return, long-term recovery will be assisted by a lessening of hydrostatic pressures (which can be achieved by elevating the fatigued body segments relative to the heart), and by enhancing the muscle pump with gentle active movements. 'Warming down' after competition has indeed a great deal to recommend it.

Recovery lag Some very short duration activities (e.g. weightlifting and pole vaulting) are characterised by a heart-rate acceleration which follows the beginning of activity but which is too slow to take much effect during the activity.[59] The heart rate continues to rise during recovery for perhaps 30 seconds or more, then exhibits the typical short- and long-duration recovery curves. Assessments of cardiac response to such activities should continue for some time post-exercise in order to catch the maximum point in the curve.

Chronic circulatory response to exercise

The function of the heart and circulation is the subject of a great number of long-term investigations, especially since it is fundamental to positive health and longevity. It is doubtful whether many first-class sportsmen are concerned with and motivated by thoughts of longevity, or even with health as a product of their training.[25] However, the pursuit of maximum performance and the enhancement of physical function does have chronic effects, and these are often used as justification for the inclusion (and sometimes the exclusion) of sports training within educational and institutional programmes.

Understandably, it is extremely difficult to structure controlled trials relating exercise to longevity and health. What can be done is to examine the chronic effects of exercise and to make assumptions about longevity and the health effects of the observed phenomena.

It is generally accepted that cardiac muscular hypertrophy and volume is proportional to the length of the competition period. Those long-distance performers whose locomotor activities cover periods in excess of one hour, of both intermittent and constant exercise, develop the largest hearts (e.g. 500 g). Such activities include team games with a great locomotor demand, such as professional soccer.[56] Proportionately smaller cardiac dimensions are observed in middle-distance athletes. In view of the high circulatory demands of events such as 1500 m run and 400 m swim this is a somewhat surprising finding, but can be explained in terms of the mechanical efficiency of the long-distance performer. The limits to long-duration aerobic function are directly linked with Vo_2 and therefore cardiac capacity. Middle-distance performers can compensate for lower cardiac capacity by greater stress tolerance. Using CAF (p. 100) as a measure of stress tolerance, middle-distance performers do record higher values (Table 3.5).[52]

TABLE 3.5   *CAF values as an indication of stress tolerance.*

	n	Mean age	Mean CAF
Middle distance sportsmen	76	20·8	35·42
Long distance sportsmen	39	23·2	34·62
Male games players	41	20·2	34·58
Male first-year PE students	135	19·8	32·80
Female first-year PE students	26	19·3	31·39
First-class sportswomen	24	22·3	33·12

There is evidence that cardiac muscle is similar to skeletal muscle in returning towards precompetitive dimensions once an athlete retires from training.[28] There is no unequivocal evidence that the heart is in any way damaged by its excursion into (and out of) the dimensions of supernormality.

With cardiac hypertrophy from training there is a proportional expansion of both the coronary vessels [47] and the capillaries.[38] The same workers have also demonstrated increases in skeletal muscular capillary volumes. The increased dimensions of the circulatory system lead to a greater economy of work *at all levels of physical work* by comparison with the untrained heart.[28] Even though the athlete experiences extreme demands on his circulation during training and competition, the lower than normal demands during rest are such that the total demands of each 24-hour period are less than normal. While he maintains circulatory fitness, therefore, the sportsman has a bigger and stronger heart, coping with a smaller total cardiac work demand.

In view of the foregoing, it is not surprising that increased circulatory damage is not to be discovered in high performance athletes of advanced age.[62]

A third category is of middle-aged relatively sedentary persons, who begin athletic training late in life. Vo_2max increases in these cases.[20] The authors stated that the increase was not due to increased a–v oxygen difference or maximum heart rate, but to an increase in stroke volume *without* a concomitant increase in heart volume. There was, therefore an increase in ventricular emptying. Other workers [7, 14, 30, 46, 51] have discovered that older sedentary persons who are exposed to physical conditioning experience cardiac hypertrophy, diminished heart rate, increased Vo_2max and increased a–v oxygen difference.

In view of this evidence there is little doubt that with correct training and competition, not only is the older sportsman unlikely to suffer circulatory damage, but also he is likely to withstand the ill effects of ageing far better than his sedentary peers.

Functional abnormalities

In one sense, the sportsman's circulatory function can be termed totally abnormal since his very existence is so different from the ordinary sedentary person. What has been discussed previously in this chapter can be regarded more as a development of normal function. There are other changes however which differ in nature from normal function.

A common abnormality is the occurrence of extra or lost beats during extreme performance (Fig. 3.18). These are due to the sportsman's heart having difficulty in coping with the

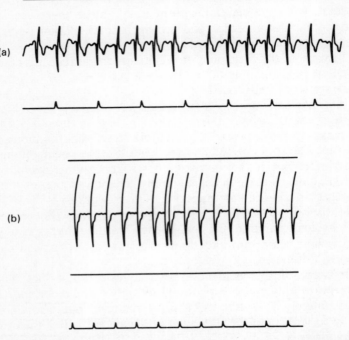

Fig. 3.18 (a) Lost beats and (b) gained beats during exercise electrocardiography

heavy demands being placed upon it. They represent attempts to catch up with a mounting demand, or to rest from the embarrassing load, and may occur during work or the recovery period. Though indicative of a lower than desirable efficiency of circulation such abnormalities ought not to be seen as pathologic [26] and were generally regarded as acceptable abnormalities by many workers at the World Congress

of Sports Medicine in 1966. The Russian sports scientist
Letounov regards extra systoles as being indicative of
dystrophy of the heart musculature caused by physical over
exertion.[32]

 A third abnormality is seen in the fluctuations in rhythm of
the heart during maximal or submaximal competition (Fig.
3.19). This represents a control hunting for the correct heart

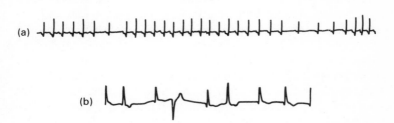

(a)

(b)

Fig. 3.19 (a) Rhythmic and (b) non-rhythmic heart rate fluctuations during exercise

rate, very common in many physical functions. The phenomenon has not been demonstrated to be pathologic in sportsmen.

Experiments in circulatory function

Since much organic function during exercise and competition
is inaccessible to even the most sophisticated of investigations, the heart rate tends to be the most widely used parameter in sports science. Nevertheless, it is still important to
ensure the validity or reliability of the heart rate as a measure.
When being used as an indicator of steady state response to
exercise or rest, lengthy periods of pulse counting are necessary — certainly not less than a minute, where possible. Where
transient responses are being monitored a shorter time is
more suitable — 5 seconds or less. It is often more convenient
to count a certain number of pulses (say 10), but account
should be taken of the shortening of the time period as the rate

increases. In some highly specific situations a beat by beat analysis is preferred, though each beat can be expressed as a rate per minute if desired.[1] Temporal fluctuations in segments of the cardiac cycle are well worthy of investigation using an electrocardiograph. Estimates of exercise heart rate may be made from post-exercise rates, using equations from Table 3.4.

Referring to p. 248 for a reminder of suitable experimental construction, the student is advised that parameters may be divided into certain subgroups. One or more items from each group may be examined in one experiment, with all groups being investigated or one or more groups held constant during the experiment. Where constancy cannot be assured, assumptions about fluctuations may be made by referring to standard texts and their descriptions of such fluctuations. On a within subject basis (test–retest) such assumptions are less critical.

Work level:

(a) ergometer – cycle, rowing, running;
(b) mechanical – weight moved × distance per unit time;
(c) performance – lap times, jumps or steps made;
(d) subjective – fatigue feelings;
(e) tactical – playing position, doubles v singles, type of play.

Circulatory response:

(a) heart rate – absolute or proportional;
(b) blood pressure – absolute or proportional;
(c) oxygen uptake ⎫
(d) carbon dioxide production ⎬ respiratory;
(e) arterio-venous oxygen difference ⎱ direct or by
(f) stroke volume ⎰ inference.

Environment:

(a) temperature;
(b) humidity;
(c) noise;
(d) emotional stimuli;

(e) surrounding medium (air, water, clothing);
(f) barometric pressure;
(g) air mixture.

Metabolism:

(a) blood lactate;
(b) blood glucose;
(c) ingestion, particularly glucose;
(d) diurnal fluctuations.

Work type:

(a) constant;
(b) incremental;
(c) intermittent;
(d) aerobic–anaerobic;
(e) recovery (short or long);
(f) body position (erect, supine, different sports positions).

References

1. ADAM, K. (1972) Personal communication.
2. ASERINSKY, E. and KLEITMAN, N. (1953) 'Regularly occurring periods of eye motility and concomitant phenomena during sleep'. *Science*, **118**, 273.
3. ASMUSSEN, E. (1946) 'Aerobic recovery after anaerobiosis in rest and work'. *Acta physiologica scandinavica*, **11**, 197.
4. ASTRAND, I. (1960) 'Aerobic work capacity in men and women with special reference to age'. *Acta physiologica scandinavica*, **49**, Suppl., 169.
5. ASTRAND, P-O. and RHYMING, I. (1954) 'A nomogram for calculation of aerobic capacity (physical fitness) from pulse rate during submaximal work'. *Journal of Applied Physiology*, **7**, 218.
6. ASTRAND, P-O. *et al.* (1964) 'Cardiac output during maximal and submaximal work'. *Journal of Applied Physiology*, **19**, 268.
7. BAAR. (1963) 'Degenerative heart diseases from lack of exercise'. *Proceedings, College Exercise and Fitness, Illinois*.
8. BERGSTROM, J. *et al.* (1967) 'Diet, muscle glycogen and physical performance'. *Acta physiologica scandinavica*, **71**, 140.
9. BERGSTROM, J. and HULTMAN, E. (1967) 'A study of the glycogen

metabolism during exercise in man'. *Scandinavian Journal of Clinical and Laboratory Investigation*, **19**, 218.

10. BEVEGARD, S. *et al.* (1963) 'Circulatory studies in well trained athletes'. *Acta physiologica scandinavica*, **57**, 26.

11. BROOKE, J. D. *et al.* (1968) 'Relationship of the heart rate to physical work'. *Proceedings of the Physiological Society*, April.

12. BROUHA, L. (1943) 'The step test: a simple method of measuring physical fitness for muscular work in young men'. *Research Quarterly of the American Association for Health, Physical Education and Welfare*, **14**, 1, 31.

13. CHRISTENSEN, E. H. and HOGBERG, P. (1950) 'The efficiency of anaerobic work'. *Arbeitsphysiologie*, **14**, 249.

14. CURETON, T. K. (1963) 'Anatomical, physiological, and psychological changes induced by exercise programs in adults'. *Proceedings, College Exercise and Fitness, Illinois.*

15. CORSER, T. and THOMAS, V. (1970) 'A study of trampoline exercise by synchronised cinephotography and electromyography'. *British Journal of Sports Medicine*, **5**, 1.

16. EKBLOM, B. *et al.* (1968) 'Effect of training on circulatory response to exercise'. *Journal of Applied Physiology*, **24**, 518.

17. GRIMBY, G., HÄGGENDAL, E. and SALTIN, B. (1967) 'Local xenon 133 clearance from the quadriceps muscle during exercise in man'. *Journal of Applied Physiology*, **22**, 305.

18. GUYTON, A. C. (1969) *Function of the human body.* W. B. Saunders: London.

19. HAMLEY, E. J. and THOMAS, V. (1967) 'Physiological and postural factors in the calibration of the bicycle ergometer'. *Journal of Physiology*, **191**, 55P.

20. HARTLEY, H. L. *et al.* (1969) 'Physical training in sedentary middle-aged and older men. Cardiac output and gas exchange at submaximal and maximal levels'. *Scandinavian Journal of Clinical and Laboratory Investigation*, **24**, 335.

21. HENDERSON, F. (1927) 'The efficiency of the heart and the significance of rapid and slow pulse rates'. *American Journal of Physiology*, 512.

22. HERMANSEN, L. *et al.* (1967) 'Muscle glycogen during prolonged severe exercise'. *Acta physiologica scandinavica*, **71**, 129.

23. HERMANSEN, L. and SALTIN, B. (1969) 'Oxygen uptake during maximal treadmill and bicycle exercise'. *Journal of Applied Physiology*, **1**, 3, 234.

24. HERMANSEN, L. (1969) 'Anaerobic energy release'. *Medicine and Science in Sports*, **1**, 1, 32.

25. HUNT, J. H. (1965) *Accident prevention and life saving.* Livingstone: London.

26. HYMAN, A. S. (1959) 'The cardiac athlete, some observations concerning functional capacity in health and disease'. *Medicina sportiva*, **13**, 313.

27. IKAI, M. *et al.* (1966) 'Physiological significance of endurance in distance and marathon runners'. *Journal of Sports Medicine and Physical Fitness*, **6**, 3, 158.

28. ISRAEL, S. (1968) 'Sports, Herzgrösse und Kreislaufdynamik'. *Sportmedizin Schriftenreihe*, 3. Leipzig.

29. ISSEKUTZ, B. *et al.* (1962) 'Use of respiratory quotients in assessment of aerobic work capacity'. *Journal of Applied Physiology*, **17**, 47.

30. JOKL, E. (1964) *Alter und Leistung.* Springer Verlag: Berlin.

31. LETOUNOV, S. P. and MOTYLYANSKAYA, R. E. (1951) *Medical control in physical education.* Fis: Moscow.

32. LETOUNOV, S. P. (1957) *Electrocardiographic and roentgenographic investigations of the sportsman's heart.* Moscow.

33. LINZBACH, A. J. (1947) 'Mikrometrische und histologische Analyse hypertropher menschlicher Herzen'. *Virchows Archiv für pathologische Anatomie und Physiologie und für klinische Medizin*, **314**, 534.

34. MARGARIA, R. *et al.* (1965) 'Indirect determination of maximum O_2 consumption in man'. *Journal of Applied Physiology*, **20**, 1070.

35. MARITZ, J. S. *et al.* (1961) 'A practical method of estimating an individual's maximal oxygen intake'. *Ergonomics*, **4**, 97.

36. MELLEROWICZ, H. (1956) 'Vergleichende Untersuchungen uber das Okonomieprincip in Arbeit und Leistung des trainierten Kreislaufs'. *Archiv für Kreislaufforschung*, **24**, 70.

37. MUSSHOFF, K. *et al.* (1959) 'Stroke volume, a–v difference, cardiac output and physical working capacity, and their relationships to heart volume'. *Acta cardiologica*, **4**, 427.

38. PETREN, T. *et al.* (1936) 'Der Einfluss des Trainings auf die Häufigkeit der Capillaren in Herz- und Skelettmuskelatur'. *Arbeitsphysiologie*, **9**, 376.

39. PROKOP, L. (1957) 'Grosserer Überlebenschance körperlich Aktiver'. *Sportphysiologie, Sportmedizin, Schriftenreihe*, Bern.

40. REINDELL, H. *et al.* (1960) *Herzkreislaufkrankheiten und Sport.* Munchen.

41. ROWELL, L. B. (1962) *Factors affecting the prediction of the maximal oxygen intake* . . . Ph.D. diss., University of Minnesota.

42. ROZENBLATT, V. V. *et al.* (1966) 'Biotelemetric observations in sports medicine'. *Proceedings of the 16th Weltkongress für Sportmedizin, Hanover.*

43. SALTIN, B. (1964) 'Circulatory response to maximal and submaximal exercise after thermal dehydration'. *Journal of Applied Physiology*, **19**, 1125.

44. SALTIN, B. and ASTRAND, P-O. (1967) 'Maximal oxygen uptake in athletes'. *Journal of Applied Physiology*, **23**, 353.

45. SALTIN, B. *et al.* (1968) 'Response to exercise after bed rest and after training'. *Circulation*, **38**, Suppl. 7, 1.

46. SARKIZOV-SERAZINI (1962) *Physical culture in advanced age*. Moscow.

47. SCHOENMAKERS, J. (1949) 'Die Herzkrankädern bei der arteriocardialen Hypertrophie'. *Z. Kreislauf. Vorsch.*, **38**, 321.

48. SJOSTRAND, T. (1947) 'Changes in respiratory organs of workmen at an ore smelting works'. *Acta medica scandinavica*, **131**, Suppl., 196.

49. SPROULE, B. J. *et al.* (1960) 'Cardiopulmonary physiological responses to heavy exercise in patients with anaemia'. *Journal of Clinical Investigation*, **39**, 378.

50. STAINSBY, W. N. and WELCH, H. G. (1966) 'Lactate metabolism of contracting dog skeletal muscle *in situ*'. *American Journal of Physiology*, **211**, 177.

51. TCHEBOTAREV, D. F. *et al.* (1965) *Physical culture – a source of longevity*. Publishing House of Physical Culture and Sport: Moscow.

52. THOMAS, V. (1971) *The tolerance of extreme physical stress in sportsmen*. Ph.D. thesis, University of Surrey.

53. THOMAS, V. (1968) 'Supermen under stress'. *New Scientist*, Oct., 40.

54. THOMAS, V. and GREEN, L. F. (1971) 'Some effects of glucose syrup ingestion during work of differing intensities and durations'. *Proceedings of the Nutrition Society*, **31**, 5a.

55. THOMAS, V. (1971) 'The effects of glucose syrup ingestion on extended locomotor performance'. *British Journal of Sports Medicine*, **5**, 4.

56. THOMAS, V. (1973) Unpublished observations.

57. THOMAS, V. (1971) *Sport and science*. Faber: London.

58. THOMAS, V. (1970) 'A test of cardiac function during strenuous exercise'. *Proceedings of the 18th World Congress on Sports Medicine*.

59. THOMAS, V. (1969) *Physiological analyses of sports performance*. M.Sc. thesis, University of Loughborough.

60. TUTTLE, W. W. and SALIT, E. P. (1945) 'The relation of resting heart rate to the increase in rate due to exercise'. *American Heart Journal*, **29**, 594.

61. WAHLUND, H. (1948) 'Determination of the physical working capacity'. *Acta medica scandinavica*, **132**, Suppl., 215.

62. WIELE, G. (1952) 'Früh- und Aufbrauchschaden des Kreislaufs beim Schwerarbeiter'. *Neuheiten auf dem Fortbildungslehrgang*, **17**, 56.

CHAPTER FOUR
Respiration

Some difficulties arise in students' minds over the meaning of the words ventilation and respiration. In this text, *ventilation* represents the mechanical process of moving volumes of air into and out of the lungs. Respiration, on the other hand, refers to the movement of individual gases from the air to the working tissues and their return via the blood, a process which *includes* ventilation.

Respiration

To a certain extent tissue respiration has been covered during the preceding chapter in what may be termed systemic respiration, resulting in arterio-venous differences of both oxygen and carbon dioxide. Now comes an examination of pulmonary respiration, which virtually reverses the effect in the long term.

Upon reaching the lungs, the pulmonary artery spreads into capillaries covering the pulmonary membrane, an extremely thin ($0 \cdot 3$ micron) membrane covering all small ventilatory vessels up to and including the respiratory bronchioles. The total area of this membrane is approximately 60 m^2 in the normal adult, and is considerably greater in sportsmen. The total blood in the pulmonary capillaries is extended to a level of 1 ml/m^2, and is therefore given great exposure to the lung air. The extent and thinness of the pulmonary membrane facilitate very efficient gas exchange in the lungs.

The transfer of gases through the pulmonary membrane takes place by diffusion and is a function of the differing pressures of the gases on either side of the membrane. The process is described in Chapter 1. Carbon dioxide diffuses twenty times more easily than oxygen being far more soluble in the fluids of the pulmonary membrane.

As described in Chapter 2, the alveolar oxygen combines mainly with the haemoglobin in the blood (Fig. 4.1). The proportion of haemoglobin holding oxygen is directly related to the pressure of oxygen, as may be seen from the standard oxygen haemoglobin dissociation curve (Fig. 4.2).

At a normal aeration level, blood leaves the lungs with an oxygen pressure of 100 mmHg, which means that about 97 per cent of the haemoglobin is combined with oxygen. Normally, therefore, the blood is virtually *fully oxygenated* in the lungs.

During resting levels, the uptake of oxygen by the tissues is such as to reduce the blood oxygen pressure to about 40 mmHg. Reference to the dissociation curve will show that

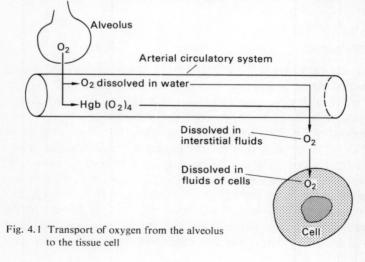

Fig. 4.1 Transport of oxygen from the alveolus
to the tissue cell

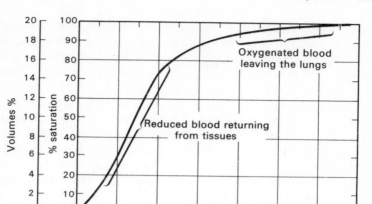

Fig. 4.2 The oxygen–haemoglobin dissociation curve

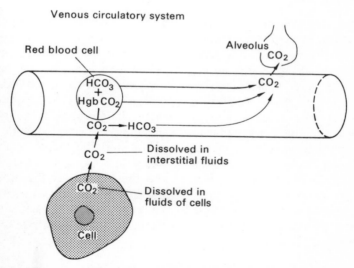

Fig. 4.3 Transport of carbon dioxide from the tissue cell to the alveolus, illustrating some of the chemical combinations of carbon dioxide with blood

only 70 per cent of the haemoglobin is combined with oxygen at that pressure, so nearly 30 per cent of the haemoglobin gives up its oxygen. During extreme levels of oxygen uptake in sport, particularly regarding the virtual exhaustion of capillary oxygen in the working muscles, as much as 90 per cent of the haemoglobin may release its oxygen. This represents a three-fold increase in oxygen supply without an increase in cardiac output. However, the healthy heart also increases its output with increased tissue demand, as described in Chapter 3.

To complete the picture, the carbon dioxide transport follows a route almost the reverse of that taken by oxygen (Fig. 4.3), except that haemoglobin is not the main carrier (Chapter 3, p. 69). The carbon dioxide pressure of the blood leaving the peripheral tissues is about 45 mmHg, which is only 5 mmHg higher than that of alveolar air. However, the rapid diffusion rate of carbon dioxide ensures that virtual equilibrium is reached in the pulmonary capillaries.

Ventilation

Ventilation is achieved via the ventilatory passages (Fig. 4.4). The forces which move the air may be described as active and passive, and are due normally to muscular effort, gravity and tissue elasticity. Occasionally, external forces may be present, e.g. in water sports, from violent physical contact and from artificial respiration. The forces normally act on the thoracic cavity (or pleural cavity), comprising the sternum, spine, rib cage and diaphragm muscle. The lungs are covered with a membrane called the visceral pleura, and the inside of the pleural cavity with the parietal pleura. The surfaces of these two membranes are lubricated and the lungs may therefore slide freely within the cavity. The gap between the two pleura is sealed, and any tendency of the lungs to become detached from the pleural cavity is resisted since it would give rise to a negative pressure.

Inspiration Enlargement of the thoracic cavity can be caused by contraction of the diaphragm and the external

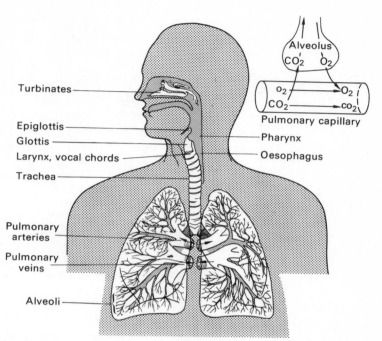

Turbinates

Epiglottis
Glottis
Larynx, vocal chords
Trachea

Pulmonary
arteries

Pulmonary
veins

Alveoli

Alveolus
CO_2 O_2

O_2 O_2
CO_2 CO_2
Pulmonary capillary

Pharynx
Oesophagus

Fig. 4.4 The respiratory system, showing the respiratory passages and function of
the alveolus to oxygenate the blood and to remove carbon dioxide

intercostal muscles, together with a relaxation of the
abdominal and internal intercostal muscles (Fig. 4.5). These
actions are active, resulting in an increased thoracic cavity
volume and a tendency to a pressure drop within the lungs. If
the airways are open, air will flow into the lungs. During
extreme rates of ventilation, athletes may consciously or
unconsciously use accessory muscles of inspiration, viz.
scaleni, sternomastoids and spinal extensors.[6]

Expiration   At the end of inspiration energy has been stored
in the elastic tissues of the lungs, thorax and stretched expiratory muscles. Elastic recoil is then sufficient to accomplish
quiet expiration, with little or no involvement of the expiratory muscles (abdominals and internal intercostals). This is

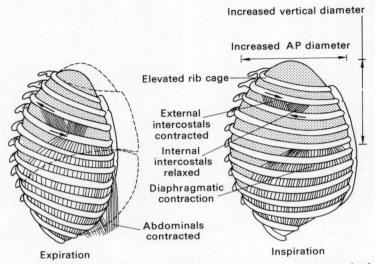

Increased vertical diameter

Increased AP diameter

Elevated rib cage

External
intercostals
contracted

Internal
intercostals
relaxed

Diaphragmatic
contraction

Abdominals
contracted

Expiration

Inspiration

Fig. 4.5 The major muscles of expiration and inspiration, and changes in the
thoracic cage during expiration and inspiration

passive expiration. At greater levels of ventilation during
exercise the expiratory musculature is brought more strongly
into play, particularly towards the end of expiration. In events
where controlled ventilation is advisable or necessary (particularly in swimming) the holding of deep inspiration imposes a greater and perhaps more explosive demand on the
expiratory muscles.

In some events the ventilatory system can be used as a
transmitter of force or as an absorber of stresses. This is
particularly true in weightlifting where abdominal and thoracic pressure changes have been recorded in the order of 250
mmHg.[11]

Ventilation volumes

Figure 4.6 shows the type of chart which may be obtained
from a spirograph recording the volumes of air entering and
leaving the lungs at different levels of exercise, and during
maximal inspiration and expiration.

Tidal volume (*VT*)   During quiet breathing, approximately 500 ml of air — called the tidal volume — is taken per breath. With a resting breathing rate of approximately 12 per minute, the minute tidal volume is 6 litres.

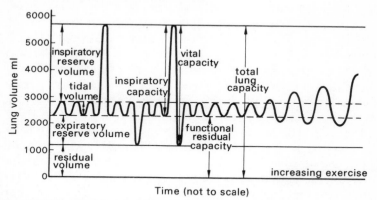

Fig. 4.6 Spirogram of various divisions of the ventilatory air

Inspiratory capacity   After inspiring the tidal volume, the sportsman may continue with a maximal inhalation. This quantity is known as the inspiratory capacity, and is normally about 3·5—4 l in a first-class athlete.

Expiratory reserve volume   After expiring the tidal volume, the sportsman may continue with a maximum exhalation. This quantity is known as the expiratory reserve volume, and is normally about 1·5 l in a first-class athlete.

Functional residual capacity (*FRC*)   After exhalation at any stage of exercise there is a volume of air remaining within the airways, composed of the unused portion of expiratory reserve volume, and a volume of air which it is impossible to exhale called the residual volume — normally about 1·5 l. This air permits some gaseous exchange to proceed in the alveoli between inspirations. Within the airways themselves there is a portion of the inspired air which cannot contribute to gas exchange since it is not in contact with pulmonary capillaries.

This is the dead space and amounts to about 150–200 ml. During low levels of ventilation, the dead space forms a large part of the ventilation volume. For example, of 500 ml tidal volume, only 350 ml of that new air will contact the alveoli. It has been shown that dead space can double during heavy exercise.[3] During rest, the 350 ml of new air entering the alveoli mixes with the FRC which may be as much as 2 l. Each breath, then, may change only $\frac{1}{6}$ of the alveolar air, which ensures that the constituents of alveolar air do not fluctuate too rapidly. At higher levels of ventilation during competition (say 130 l/min, with approximately 60 per cent of vital capacity being used) the tidal volume would be about 3 l, mixing with the FRC of 2 l. In this case, $\frac{2}{3}$ of the alveolar air can be refreshed with new air per breath. Hyperventilation can flush alveolar air rapidly, and is a standard technique for divers wishing to depress their blood carbon dioxide levels for prolonged immersion – or to clear rapidly oxygen deficit after immersion. It is also a dangerous technique since it tampers with a breathing response which may be critical in deep diving, this response being sensitive to blood carbon dioxide levels. The implications for subaquatic sports are obvious, particularly in snorkel activities and games such as octopush.

Vital capacity (*VC*)   From maximum inspiration to maximum expiration is called the vital capacity – the total quantity of air which can be moved into and out of the lungs. Though the average vital capacity of first-class athletes is not much larger than normal (5 litres against 4·5 litres), some sportsmen have extremely large lungs, and values of over 7 litres are not uncommon. The vital capacity is closely related to body build, race, altitude of domicile, habitual exercise, smoking, sex, etc. As an individual predictor of fitness it might not therefore be considered to be particularly reliable. However, it has been discovered to be one of the better fitness indices in a heterogeneous sports population,[35] and has the advantage of being an easily measured factor. Some studies which show vital capacities of good-class sportsmen to be no different from average and unrelated to ability were per-

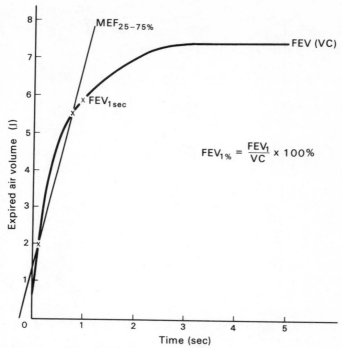

Fig. 4.7 Single breath spirogram, measured on the author

formed on a group of marathon runners,[14] a hardly surprising result in view of the demands of that activity and the typical stature of the competitors.

Pulmonary mid-capacity (MC)   At any level of ventilation, the average between the end volumes of inspiration and expiration is called the mid-capacity.

In the analysis of ventilation during performance, rates of airflow are of greater importance than absolute lung volumes. A curve of volume against time can be drawn during a single forceful exhalation (Fig. 4.7). The slope of the curve indicates lung power at any given time. Apart from the value of absolute power at given points of the curve, most commonly expressed as forced expiratory volume against time (e.g.

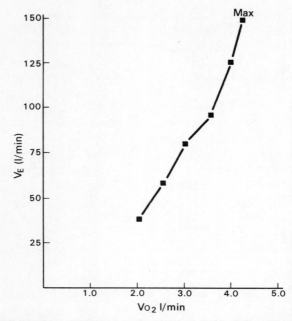

Fig. 4.8 Relationship between oxygen uptake and ventilation in well-trained sportsmen

FEV_{1sec}), proportionate measures are most useful where differences in body size should be ignored. Of these FEV expressed as a percentage of VC ($FEV_{1\%}$) and mid-expiratory flow within the second and third quarters of VC ($MEF_{25-75\%}$) are the most meaningful to sportsmen. Large scale studies have not yet been performed to derive norms for sportsmen, but it would be expected that good standard athletes should have an $FEV_{1\%}$ of between 75 and 85 per cent and an MEF of 5–7 l/min. It is noticeable that some athletes with larger lungs experience greater difficulty in exhaling a specific proportion (say 80 per cent) in an $FEV_{1\%}$. Greater values of $FEV_{1\%}$ are not necessarily indicative of better ventilation.

Minute volumes Figure 4.8 shows the curve of increasing ventilation rate (VE) with increasing V_{O_2}. It can be seen that in these sportsmen (though a similar but lower curve exists for normals), as V_{O_2} nears its asymptote, VE continues to rise. At the upper limits of sports function, increased ventilation is not associated with increased oxygen uptake. The limits to respiration are provided by the circulation rather than the ventilation. VE increases with increasing work load well into the anaerobic phases of endurance, and never reaches levels which approximate to the individual's maximum voluntary ventilation power (MVV). It has been estimated that the maximal possible ventilation during exercise is approximately 170 l/min,[24] though higher values in excess of 200 l/min have been recorded on a high performance athlete.[17] MVV in such cases can exceed 250 l/min. Later investigations of very big international basketballers have revealed VCs of 7–9 l, and MVVs of 350 l/min.

Energy cost of ventilation

Since the ventilatory muscles perform the work of breathing, some part of the V_{O_2} must be utilised in maintaining these muscles. At rest the oxygen cost of breathing is approximately 0·5 ml O_2 per litre of ventilated air – that is, around 1 per cent of the total metabolic cost. Trained sportsmen can maintain this 1 per cent cost up to approximately 75 per cent of their maximum aerobic work rate, but beyond that point the proportion of oxygen going to the working muscles increases rapidly to values as high as 7 per cent,[25] 9 per cent[28] and 20 per cent.[29] If the ventilatory muscles are taking an increased proportion of the V_{O_2}max, then there is less remaining for the locomotor musculature. The precise debits and credits of the balance of V_{O_2}max power have not been evaluated for sportsmen, but it is clear that increases in ventilation above the aerobic level are undesirable on two counts;

(1) increasing demands on available oxygen;
(2) increased feelings of ventilatory distress may inhibit increased performance.[19]

Flow resistances

The importance of blood vessel resistances was mentioned in Chapter 3. Similar effects are noticeable for air flow within the ventilatory tracts. The difficulties of evaluating resistances which are meaningful for the sportsman are highlighted by the finding that the oxygen cost of ventilation at a given rate in a comfortable arm chair is about 70 per cent of the cost of the same ventilation rate while riding a bicycle. The compliance of the air tracts does not rival that of the blood vessels. Increases in fluid flow in the airways result in dramatic increases in flow resistances provided by:

(1) tissue elasticity in lungs and bony thorax: 20 per cent;
(2) airway and tissue friction resistances ⎫ 80 per cent.
(3) inertia of gases and moving tissues ⎭

Since the resistance to nasal breathing is up to three times that to oral breathing, the latter is preferred even in events of low ventilation.

Mechanics of ventilation

A chart of tidal volumes expressed as percentages of vital capacity at different levels of exercise on a bicycle, with different rates of spontaneous breathing, demonstrates that the augmentation of minute ventilation is achieved mainly by an increase in ventilation rate and the use of inspiratory capacity (Fig. 4.9).[15]

The contribution of the thoracic cage can be examined in comparison with that of the abdomen during exercise ventilation at different levels. It can be seen that, whereas at resting the contribution of the abdominal wall is small but positive, during light work (44 l/min VE) the abdominal contribution decreases and becomes negative, a change which is even more accentuated during fairly heavy work on a bicycle (130 l/min VE). If, however, such levels of ventilation are voluntarily performed during seated rest, the fall in abdominal contribution is not present.[11] It is probable, therefore, that at least

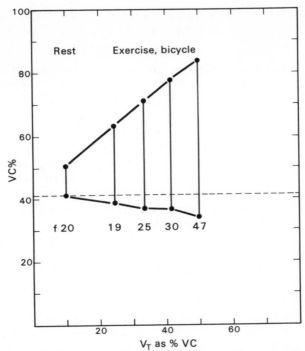

Fig. 4.9 End-inspiratory and end-expiratory values (vertical axes) at different tidal volumes, expressed as % of vital capacity (horizontal axes).[15] The respiratory rates are given

during hard cycling the abdominal work of breathing is diverted elsewhere, possibly in synergic or fixator work for leg pedalling movements.

Effects of altitude on respiration

The siting of major sporting events at high altitude (e.g. Mexico City – 2300 m), and the superiority of some athletes who have lived or trained at high altitudes, has caused much sports scientific attention to be focused on respiratory responses to altitude. The main physiological response is to the decrease in barometric pressure, since this depresses the pressure of oxygen in the air, the alveoli, and so the arterial oxygen saturation.

Altitude	Barometric pressure	Oxygen pressure in air	Oxygen pressure in alveoli	Arterial oxygen saturation
metres	mmHg	mmHg	mmHg	%
0	760	159	104	97
3000	523	110	67	90

It can well be imagined that a decrease in arterial oxygen saturation of 7 per cent is most critical to performers who require high aerobic levels – at an altitude of 6000 m a decrease of 27 per cent is experienced, which of course spells a metaphorical death knell for most competitors, and occasionally actual death for mountaineers.

Sportsmen accustomed to training and competing at low altitudes will experience an automatic hyperventilation on ascending to high altitude. This hyperventilation is due to low oxygen pressures in arterial blood [1, 4] rather than to high carbon dioxide pressures (the latter being depressed by the hyperventilation). The decrease in total blood carbon dioxide leads to the excretion of bicarbonate in order to maintain normal blood acidity, which causes a decrease in plasma volume *but not* an overall decrease in haemoglobin.[2] After a period of acclimatisation lasting from one to several weeks, the plasma volume returns to normal and an increase in haemoglobin can be observed. Permanent residents at high altitude may develop red blood cell counts of 50 per cent more than is normal at sea level.

In considering briefly the effects on different events of competing at altitude, a subdivision is necessary.

Sub-V$o_2$max events: The very long distance events such as 20 km walk, the marathon and cycling road race. The evidence suggests that the oxygen cost of these events is similar to that at sea level.[9, 22, 30] With a reduced alveolar oxygen pressure and arterial oxygen saturation, an equivalent Vo_2 can be achieved only by increasing cardiac output and ventilation rate. In fact during the first week or so, cardiac output may increase by up to 60 per cent for a given submaximal work load, then returning slowly to previous (sea-level) values.[2, 8, 22, 36] Also, the ventilation rate increases at given work rates (Fig. 4.10).

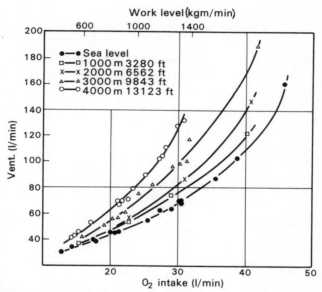

Fig. 4.10 Pulmonary ventilation in relation to oxygen uptake at different work levels when breathing air at acute exposure to various simulated altitudes up to 4000 m (Astrand, P-O.: *Acta physiol. scand.*, **30**, 1954)

It is clear, then, that sub-V_{O_2}max events *could* proceed at the same pace as at sea level provided the competitors could tolerate an elevated ventilation rate and maintain an increased cardiac output. If the previous limits to their performance had been of locomotor muscular efficiency and endurance, it is possible that high altitude would not pose insuperable problems of maintaining work output – unless the oxygen dissociation at the working tissues was affected (which is likely in view of the decreased arterial oxygen pressure).

Performances at the Mexico Olympics showed such a falling off as to make it virtually certain that the total respiratory function suffers during competition at high altitude, even after considerable attempts at acclimatisation.

Maximum V_{O_2} events   Most track events excluding short sprints. The limitations of maximum cardiac output with a decreased arterial oxygen pressure (and thus decreased V_{O_2} max), and of greater energy costs associated with higher ventilation rates, ensure that performances will suffer dramatically in such events. Circulo-respiratory factors at altitude are shown in Table 4.1.[5]

TABLE 4.1   *Effects of altitude on the circulatory factors involved in oxygen transport*

	Rest	Maximal work			
	sea level	sea level	2300 m	4200 m	5600 m
Heart rate (beats/min)	52	180	172	168	164
Stroke volume (ml)	100	174	174	170	150
Articular-venous O_2 difference (per cent by volume)	4·5	16	15	13	11
Oxygen intake (ml/min)	234	5000	4500	3700	2700
Max V_{O_2} (per cent of 'normal')	—	100	90	74	54

These figures show that athletes could expect a decrement of at least 10 per cent in V_{O_2}max when moving from sea level to Mexico City. This represents a definite reduction factor in performance which could not be circumvented by increased cardiac or ventilatory output – though the ventilation rate at the (lower) maximal work rate *is* higher, by approximately 25 per cent.

Maximal work (anaerobic)   It has previously been demonstrated that the medium-duration maximal work (as distinct from short-duration explosive events) deteriorates at altitude.

While the part played by depressed V_{O_2}max is clear, the effects of altitude on the competitor's ability to tolerate anaerobiosis have not been so fully investigated. Maximal blood lactate during exhaustion (at a lower work rate) shows a slighter fall than other parameters on reaching high altitude, and may even improve on sea-level standards within a few weeks.[23]

Explosive events are virtually wholly dependent on stored energy, and it seems unlikely that such stores, or their utilisation, are affected significantly by altitude. In fact, such events are likely to benefit from the decreased gravity and air resistances to be found at high altitude.

Smoking

In considering the effects of smoking upon sportsmen, it is as well to demolish old wives' tales (such as 'smoking stunts your growth') and to ignore those effects which are irrelevant to competitive performance. Certainly it has been demonstrated that mothers who smoke during their pregnancy are more likely to have smaller babies,[18, 33] and would-be jockeys are well advised to select their parents most carefully in this respect. Karpovitch states that strength and reaction time are unaffected by smoking,[21] but the inhalation of carbon monoxide allows the gas to diffuse into the blood at a concentration of up to 5 per cent.[7, 21] This carbon monoxide then inhibits the release of oxygen to the working tissues,[34] though blood pressure and heart rate increase and remain raised for 15–60 minutes after smoking. Events demanding efficient and high V_{O_2}max are therefore inhibited by smoking, but events demanding explosive power, skill or balance [12, 13] do not seem to be affected. A 25 per cent contraction in the visual field has been reported for nonsmokers after smoking for two weeks, and an improvement of 36 per cent in smokers after two weeks abstinence.[20] Smoking causes a rise in blood sugar,[26] a decrease of 50 per cent in airway conductance lasting an hour,[27] a decrease in FEV immediately after smoking [32] and a three-fold increase in respiratory tract resistance after one cigarette.

The tar deposits within the lungs of heavy smokers possibly have an effect on sportsmen, by reducing their total lung capacity. However, since the sportsman never needs his full capacity during competition, it is probable that the effect is not significant. Direct evidence of smoking in sport is pitifully thin, though investigations of superbly conditioned swimmers have shown no deleterious changes in pulmonary function immediately after smoking two cigarettes in succession.[31] There are many cases where champion sportsmen derive considerable psychophysiological benefits from smoking *an occasional* cigarette. Provided the overall consumption of cigarettes is small, there seems to be no critical athletic reason for preventing a sportsman from taking the occasional smoke, nor any firm evidence that heavy smoking is necessarily injurious to competitive performance in explosive events. The chronic effects on the sportsman's general health and longevity may, of course, be sufficient reason for encouraging him to refrain from the habit.

Subaquatic respiration

Subaquatic sports divide into two distinct categories. The first embraces activities where the participant exists on the volume of air inhaled before diving and returns to the surface for each breath. This is skin diving, with perhaps the assistance of fins, face mask, snorkel tube and wet suit. The second division is termed scuba diving (scuba being an acronym for Self-Contained Underwater Breathing Apparatus) and involves carrying a cylinder of compressed gases, with various ancillary equipment.

Skin diving

Accomplished performers may achieve depths of between 50 and 100 ft, remaining submerged for two minutes and longer.

The great involvement of the skeletal musculature in swimming itself presents considerable energy demands which, in
addition to the energy costs of respiration, may precipitate
increases in Vo_2 and carbon dioxide formation in excess of
20-fold.[16] The normal ventilatory reaction is to increase VE,
but if ventilation is withheld carbon dioxide levels in tissues
and blood increase enormously. Blood carbon dioxide is the
basic stimulus for breathing, and high levels give the swimmer
the well-known 'panic for air' feeling which eventually forces
him to the surface to breathe.

During skin diving the time of submergence is so short as
to prevent the occurrence of nitrogen narcosis, bends, gid-
diness and unconsciousness which are prevalent dangers in
scuba diving. On the other hand, descent through 10 m causes
an increase in barometric pressure of one atmosphere, which
is sufficient to compress the body gases by a half. Air which is
trapped in body cavities such as the sinus orifices, trachea,
bronchii and inner ear can transmit pressures sufficiently
great to rupture body tissues; the most common injury is a
ruptured tympanic membrane. The ears are extremely sensitive to pressure changes, and divers ought to be guided by
aural warning signals. Pressures can be relieved by swallowing or chewing movements, which tend to open the
Eustachian tubes.

Scuba diving

During the deeper diving which may be performed by scuba
divers, the blood gases are subjected to even greater pressures. These pressures particularly affect the gases, oxygen
and nitrogen, which diffuse into the blood by virtue of the
'atmospheric' pressure. The pressures of carbon dioxide in the
blood are not directly related to atmospheric pressure, and
are not directly affected by depth. At depths in excess of 60 m
the increase in oxygen pressure is such that the cellular
oxygen content becomes unbalanced, leading at progressively
greater depths to cellular damage, abnormality in function or
even death from oxygen poisoning. The danger is avoided if

the gas mixture being supplied to the diver contains progressively less oxygen.

At similar depths, the increased nitrogen pressure can have an anaesthetic effect, causing sleep or drunkenness. This possibility can be avoided by substituting helium for nitrogen in the gas supply, since helium has no effect on the body functions and diffuses out of the body very rapidly during ascent to the surface.

The most critical factor for the scuba diver is the tendency of carbon dioxide to accumulate in his face mask, with the resulting possibility of coma through respiratory acidosis. This accumulation is prevented by ensuring that a constant and sufficient volume of fresh gas is flushing the mask. Since the volume is directly proportional to the depth, and at 60 m approximately seven times as much cylinder air must be released into the mask as would be needed at surface level, the carbon dioxide washout is the controlling factor for air supply to the scuba diver.

Experiments in respiration

Experiments in this area are very much restricted by the apparatus available. Since ventilation can be so much under voluntary control, it is difficult to avoid psychological effects during experiments. Ventilation rate is relatively easy to measure, but relatively meaningless unless linked with ventilation volumes. Students also ought to be warned that measuring lung function by using face masks, nose clips, mouthpieces, etc. imposes physical and psychological loads on subjects which, in all except those very accustomed to such techniques, may cause great experimental errors.

When single breath responses are monitored, the most reliable volumetric data can be obtained from maximum functions. When monitoring nonmaximal functions, measuring periods ought to be as long as possible, thus reducing the mean error.

The reader is referred to p. 248 for a reminder of suitable

experiment construction, and is advised that parameters may be divided into certain subgroups. One or more items from each group *may* be examined on one experiment, with *all* groups being investigated or one or more groups held constant during the experiment. Where constancy cannot be assured, then assumptions about fluctuations may be made by referring to standard tests, and their descriptions of such fluctuations. On a within subjects basis (test–retest) such assumptions are less critical.

Work level:

  (a) ergometer – cycle, rowing, running, etc.;
  (b) mechanical – weight moved and distance per unit time;
  (c) performance – lap times, jumps or steps made;
  (d) subjective – fatigue feelings;
  (e) tactical – playing position, doubles *v* singles, type of play, etc.

Respiratory response:

  (a) ventilatory rate, volume, power;
  (b) oxygen uptake – proportional or absolute;
  (c) carbon dioxide production – proportional or absolute;
  (d) breath holding – time elapsed;
  (e) hypo- and hyperventilation – with care and supervision.

Environment:

  (a) temperature;
  (b) humidity;
  (c) emotional stimuli;
  (d) locomotor rhythm;
  (e) barometric pressure;
  (f) air mixture;
  (g) tobacco smoking.

Metabolism:

  (a) blood lactate;
  (b) blood glucose;
  (c) ingestion, particularly glucose;
  (d) diurnal fluctuations.

References

1. ASMUSSEN, E. and CHIODI, H. (1941) 'The effect of hypoxaemia on ventilation and circulation in man'. *American Journal of Physiology*, **132**, 426.
2. ASMUSSEN, E. and CONSOLAZIO, F. C. (1941) 'The circulation in rest and work on Mount Evans (4300 m)'. *American Journal of Physiology*, **132**, 555.
3. ASMUSSEN, E. and NIELSEN, M. (1956) 'Physiological dead space and alveolar gas pressures at rest and during muscular exercise'. *Acta physiologica scandinavica*, **38**, 1.
4. ASMUSSEN, E. and CHRISTENSEN, E. H. (1966) *Kompendiumi speciel gymnastikteorie*. University of Copenhagen.
5. BALKE, B. (1971) 'Altitude factors influencing activity'. In, *Encyclopedia of Sport Science and Medicine*. American College of Sports Medicine and Macmillan: New York.
6. CAMPBELL, E. J. M. (1957) *The respiratory muscles and the mechanics of breathing*. Lloyd Luke: London.
7. CHEVALIER, R. B. *et al.* (1966) 'Reaction of non-smokers to carbon monoxide inhalation, at rest and during exercise'. *Journal of the American Medical Association*, **198**, 1961.
8. CHRISTENSEN, E. H. and FORBES, W. H. (1937) 'Der Kreislauf in grossen Hohen'. *Skandinavisches Archiv für Physiologie*, **76**, 75.
9. CHRISTENSEN, E. H. (1937) 'Sauerstoffaufnahme und respiratorische Functionen in grossen Hohen'. *Skandinavisches Archiv für Physiologie*, **76**, 88.
10. COMROE, J. H. (1966) 'The Lung'. *Scientific American*, **214**, 56.
11. SAUNDERS, G. and THOMAS, V. (1967) Unpublished observations.
12. EDWARDS, A. S. (1942) 'The measurement of static ataxia'. *American Journal of Psychology*, **55**, 171.
13. EDWARDS, A. S. (1947) 'Body sway and non-visual factors'. *Journal of Psychology*, **23**, 241.
14. GORDON, B. *et al.* (1924) 'Observations on a group of marathon runners'. *Archives of Internal Medicine*, **33**, 425.
15. GRIMBY, G. *et al.* (1968) 'Respiratory, abdominal and rib cage mechanics during exercise and induced hyperventilation'. *XXIV International Congress of Physiological Sciences*.
16. GUYTON, A. C. (1966) 'Regulation of respiration'. In, *Textbook of Medical Physiology*. W. B. Saunders: Philadelphia.
17. HAMLEY, E. J. and THOMAS, V. (1967) Unpublished observations.
18. HERRIOT, A. *et al.* (1962) 'Cigarette smoking and pregnancy'. *Lancet*, **1**, 771.

19. HOWELL, J. B. L. and CAMPBELL, E. J. M. (1966) *Breathlessness*. Blackwell: Oxford.

20. JOHNSTON, D. M. (1965) 'Preliminary report on the effect of smoking on the size of the visual fields'. *Life Sciences*, **4**, 2215.

21. KARPOVICH, P. (1965) *Physiology of muscular activity*. W. B. Saunders: Philadelphia.

22. KLAUSEN, K. (1966) 'Man's acclimatisation to altitude during the first week at 3800 m'. *Schweizerische Zeitschrift fur Sportmedizen*, **14**, 246.

23. KLAUSEN, K. *et al.* (1966) 'Effect of high altitude on maximum working capacity'. *Journal of Applied Physiology*, **21**, 1191.

24. MARGARIA, R. *et al.* (1960) 'Mechanical work of breathing during muscular exercise'. *Journal of Applied Physiology*, **15**, 354.

25. MILIC-EMILI, J. *et al.* (1962) 'Mechanical work of breathing during exercise in trained and untrained subjects'. *Journal of Applied Physiology*, **17**, 43.

26. MURCHISON, L. E. and FYFE, T. (1966) 'Effects of cigarette smoking on serum lipids, blood glucose and platelet adhesiveness'. *Lancet*, **2**, 182.

27. NADEL, J. A. and COMROE, J. H. (1961) 'Acute effects of inhalation of cigarette smoke on airway conductance'. *Journal of Applied Physiology*, **16**, 713.

28. NIELSEN, M. (1936) 'Die Respirationsarbeit bei Körperuhe und bei Muskelarbeit'. *Skandinavisches Archiv für Physiologie*, **74**, 299.

29. OTIS, A. B. (1964) 'The work of breathing'. In, *Handbook of Physiology*, Vol. 3, Pt. 1. Washington, D.C.

30. PUGH, L. G. C. E. (1958) 'Muscular exercise on Mount Everest'. *Journal of Physiology*, **141**, 233.

31. SHAPIRO, W. and PATTERSON, J. L. (1962) 'Effects of smoking and athletic conditioning on ventilatory mechanics'. *American Review of Respiratory Diseases*, **85**, 191.

32. SIMONSSON, B. (1962) 'Effect of cigarette smoking on the forced expiratory flow rate'. *American Review of Respiratory Diseases*, **85**, 534.

33. Surgeon General's Advisory Committee on Smoking and Health (1964) *Smoking and Health*. Government Printing Office: Washington, D.C.

34. Surgeon General's Report (1967) The health consequences of smoking. Government Printing Office: Washington, D.C.

35. THOMAS, V. (1972) 'Ventilatory measures of fitness in sportsmen'. *Proceedings of the Olympic Scientific Congress, Munich, 1972*.

36. VOGEL, J. A. *et al.* (1967) 'Cardiovascular responses in man during exhaustive work at sea level and at high altitude'. *Journal of Applied Physiology*, **23**, 531.

CHAPTER FIVE

Digestion

The function of the digestive system is to provide nutrients for the body. In a wide view of sports function, the system will be considered in its major functional subdivisions:

(1) ingestion – the taking in of nutrients;
(2) absorption – the transfer of nutrient constituents to the tissues;
(3) metabolism – the use of nutrients;
(4) excretion – the removal and ejection of waste products.

Ingestion

Ingestion and excretion is a process of placing nutrients in one end (the mouth) of a long muscular tube, passing them through the tube while processing them in different ways, and pushing them out at the other end (the anus) of the tube. The ramifications, expansions and convolutions of the tube (the gastrointestinal tract) are shown in Fig. 5.1. The tract itself is basically a muscular tube lined with membranes which secrete juices to break down the food, and accept the passage of nutrients out of and waste products into the tract (Fig. 5.2).

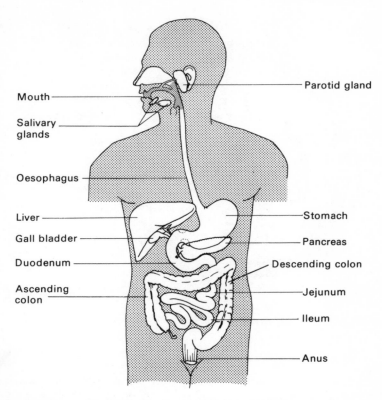

Fig. 5.1 The gastrointestinal tract from the mouth to the anus

The muscular wall of the tract performs two forms of movement:

(1) peristalsis – a slow wave-like constriction of the tract which squeezes the contents ahead of it, thus achieving their transport through the whole length of the tract. The wave travels at approximately 3 cm/second. The nervous stimulus is initiated by the first distension of the tract by food entering, and then it travels forward

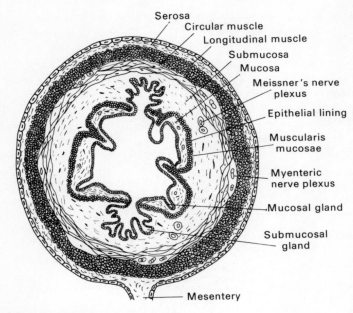

Fig. 5.2 Typical cross-section of the gut

along the tract, initiating transverse impulses at each point, causing the annular constrictions;

(2) mixing – apart from the mixing effect of peristalsis, there are rapid 'chopping' constrictions which occur at several points simultaneously, at several times a minute.

The muscles of the pharynx and of the upper oesophagus are voluntary 'skeletal' muscles. The action of swallowing is therefore a voluntary one, but is then followed by the involuntary contractions of the visceral musculature of the tract. The upper part of the stomach is an extremely distensible bag called the corpus. A large quantity of food may be held in transit here, waiting for its turn to proceed through the major absorption sections of the tract. Large quantities of gastric juices are secreted, and mixed with the food in the corpus by peristaltic and mixing waves occurring a few times a minute. By the time food reaches the lower stomach (antrum) the mixing waves are much stronger, and the food becomes a mixture called chyme which is intermittently ejected by very powerful peristalsis into the duodenum.

Within the small intestine the chyme is still continually subject to mixing waves, and is propelled gradually into the large intestine. Here the muscular movements become much less frequent since the colons are used as storage vessels. An overfilling of part of the colon leads to a strong peristalsic surge whenever necessary, even at the distal end of the descending colon. However, constriction of the external anal sphincter, which is a skeletal muscle, prevents defaecation until a desirable moment. Mixing movements occur at intervals of a few minutes, maintaining the plastic state of the faeces, and assisting the removal of water and electrolytes.

Absorption

Secretions

Nutrients are extracted from food under the action of various secretions which are made at different stages through the digestive system (Table 5.1). Mucus is secreted through all the

TABLE 5.1   *Gastrointestinal secretions*

Mouth	Stomach	Duodenum	Small intestine	Large intestine
Ptyalin (in saliva)	Hydrochloric acid Pepsin	Amylase (from pancreas) Trypsin Chymotrypsin Pancreatic lipase Sodium bicarbonate Bile (from liver)	Sucrase Maltase Lactase Pepsidases Lipases	nil

gastrointestinal tract walls, acting as lubricant to the whole system.

Digestion of carbohydrates

The constituents of carbohydrates are carbon, hydrogen and oxygen, which combine in several ways to form monosaccharides – glucose (the most common), fructose and galactose. Monosaccharides combine (polymerise) to form larger molecules such as starches and glycogen. Another carbohydrate source in the body is the disaccharides, of which maltose, sucrose and lactose are the most common. The disaccharides are formed from two molecules of monosaccharides, maltose from two glucose molecules, lactose from one of glucose and one of galactose, and sucrose from a molecule of glucose and one of fructose.

When carbohydrates are digested, the starch or other form of carbohydrate is broken down into monosaccharides. This process requires water. Enzymes in the digestive juices catalyse this process, which is called hydrolysis. The intestinal enzymes which split maltose, lactose and sucrose into their respective monosaccharides are maltase, lactase and sucrase respectively. The most abundant product of carbohydrate digestion is in fact glucose which forms 80 per cent of the glycogen stock, with galactose and fructose forming about 10 per cent each.

Carbohydrate absorption

Monosaccharides are absorbed from the intestine via the blood capillaries of the villi which project into the intestine, by a process of active absorption (see Chapter 1). They may therefore be absorbed into the bloodstream even when the intestinal concentration is very small compared with that in the blood. The fructose and galactose molecules are mostly absorbed by the liver and converted into glucose; indeed, glucose is the basis of carbohydrate metabolism in the sportsman.

The blood carries glucose to the working tissues where it enters the cell, again by active transport. The process can only take place adequately if there is enough insulin, which is the main determinant of glucose transport through the cell membrane.

The liver performs a buffering effect on blood glucose, which is maintained below a level of 130 mg per 100 ml. If a sudden intake of monosaccharides lifts the blood glucose, perhaps to 200 mg per 100 ml (hyperglycaemia), the blood flows via the liver, which stores the glucose as glycogen. When a heavy demand for glucose tends to deplete the blood glucose, the liver breaks glycogen down into glucose again and releases it to avoid very low blood glucose levels (hypoglycaemia). Other buffer mechanisms are:

(1) increased pancreatic production of insulin to allow more blood glucose to enter the muscle cells during hyperglycaemia;

(2) hypoglycaemia causes adrenal release of norepinephrine and epinephrine which, together with pancreatic glucagon hormone release, stimulates the rate of glucose release from the liver stores.

Digestion of fats

Neutral fats are similar to carbohydrates, in having a basic structure involving oxygen, carbon and hydrogen – though with a much lower proportion of oxygen. The fat molecule has a glycerol nucleus, with three fatty acid radicals attached. Some fatty acids are described as unsaturated, having fewer hydrogen atoms than the corresponding saturated acids, and are indistinguishable from other fatty acids in function except in having some structural functions in some special cells.

The digestion of fats is catalysed by enzymes – the lipases – which are secreted in the stomach and small intestine, and also by the pancreas. Bile salts are necessary in order to break the globules of fat into much smaller pieces for the lipase to contact. The initial digestion is into fatty acids, glycerol and glycerides, but as soon as these products have passed through the villi they reform into the original state within the lymphatic vessels. From the lymphatic vessels they pass via the thoracic duct into the bloodstream at the jugular vein.

The neutral fats then become deposited in the liver, or in special fat tissue which may exist in any body spaces. The function of these tissues is to act as an energy store, and they are readily available as fuel for many kinds of competitive activity. The turnover of fat stored in fat tissue is quite rapid, 50 per cent of it being replaced every week or so.

Fat transfer from storage to working muscles is achieved by the fat splitting under the enzymatic action of lipoprotein lipase into nonesterified fatty acids and glycerol. The nonesterified fatty acids are a combination of the fatty acid with a plasma protein called albumin. Blood fatty acids are an extremely available energy source, easily released and transported in times of energy need.

Fat can be synthesised within the liver from protein and, mainly, from glucose which is surplus to requirements or for which insufficient insulin is available to permit entrance to the cell. An excess of any food can therefore be stored as body fat.

Digestion of proteins

Proteins are formed of combinations of amino acids, of which there are twenty-three different types in the body. Thirteen of these can be internally synthesised from other amino acids; the other ten, which must be in the dietary intake, are called the essential amino acids. The digestion of protein proceeds in a similar fashion to carbohydrates and fats, beginning with the action of pepsinogen which is secreted in the stomach and forms pepsin upon contacting stomach hydrochloric acid. The protein yields polypeptides in the stomach and also proteoses and peptones, which after entering the small intestine are further split by trypsin and chymotrypsin into polypeptides. The last stage of digestion into amino acids is achieved by the peptides of the intestinal and pancreatic juices. The absorption of amino acids into the blood stream is virtually the same process as for monosaccharides.

The major function of amino acids are:

(1) to provide most of the structural materials for the cells;

(2) to form special function materials (fibrinogen, albumin, globulin);

(3) to form special chemical necessities (adenine, creatine, haem, glutamine, etc.);

(4) to provide energy, after being deaminated in the liver. The amino radicals lost in this process eventually combine with CO_2 to form urea which is excreted via the kidneys in urine;

(5) conversion to fats or carbohydrates (the fate of most excess protein).

During extreme long-duration energy expenditure and/or starvation, the energy for cellular function is derived from carbohydrates and fats. When these sources become depleted, amino acids may be mobilised, deaminated and deployed as necessary. But this process is a last ditch affair since, if it proceeds unchecked, it is the precursor of functional incapacity and death.

Liver function

The function of the liver is sufficiently important to warrant its own circulatory system (Fig. 5.3). This system ensures that blood goes direct from the intestines to the liver, before entering the general circulation. The liver functions firstly as a cleanser of the blood, removing virtually all bacteria which may have entered via the gut. Of greatest interest to the sportsman is the liver's function as a nutrient buffer. After ingestion of carbohydrates, the level of glucose in the portal blood may as much as double from 90 mg per 100 ml to 180–200 mg per 100 ml. The liver will remove and store up to 70 per cent of this excess, releasing it at times of greater

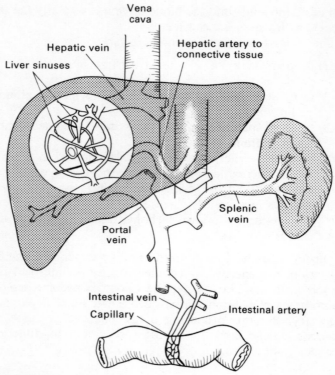

Fig. 5.3 The portal circulation

need and thus maintaining a normal level of 90–120 mg per 100 ml. This removal of glucose is accomplished by absorption through the cell membranes with the influence of insulin, conversion into glycogen and storage up to a maximum concentration of 5 g per cent of liver mass. The liver has, then, a normal maximum storage capacity of 100 g of glycogen so formed – which compares with a *normal* muscle glycogen storage capacity of 400 g. Any further excesses of portal glucose are extracted by the liver, converted into fats and sent via the circulation to storage depots in adipose tissue. During severe exercise, the liver may release sufficient glucose to contribute up to about 15 per cent of the total metabolic rate.

Protein digestion also results in amino acids entering the portal blood. The liver again acts as a buffer, extracting the amino acids to maintain blood concentration at about 30 mg per 100 ml. The amino acids combine together to be stored as small protein molecules. These may be used to synthesise fat for storage in adipose tissue.

The liver has the further nutrient function of converting non-glucose monosaccharides into glucose, while glucose may remain within the portal blood. Rapid assimilation of ingested carbohydrates in sport, therefore, is best achieved with glucose since it does not first have to undergo the conversion process.

Metabolism

In a text devoted to the physiological implications of training and competition in sports, digestion may be regarded as a fuelling and servicing system for the human machine. Having seen how the main fuels enter the body, consideration must now be given to the quantitative and qualitative uses of these fuels.

Fairly sophisticated studies of energy usage need to be made on activities which can be undertaken in a standard way near to measuring apparatus. For this reason, basic locomotor activities have been mainly used — particularly walking, running, vertical stepping and cycle pedalling. These particular locomotor modes are not only fairly common and well known to all likely subjects, but also there are stationary exercise machines and ergometers for them which enable quite precise measurements of work to be made. These are the treadmill (with incline mechanism), cycle ergometer and step or staircase (moving if possible). The 1970s have seen the emergence of reliable rowing, swimming and whole body ergometers, and there is no doubt that investigations into other locomotor modes will now proliferate.

Walking   The energy cost of walking at fairly low speeds (3—6·5 k.p.h.), of the order of speed a games player might use during quiet phases in the game for perhaps a considerable part of the game,[29] may be expressed by the equation $C = 0.8V + 0.5$, where C represents the energy expenditure in calories per minute and V the velocity in k.p.h.[22] This is a rectilinear relationship, whereas analysis of a greater range of walking speeds and inclines shows the relationship to be curvilinear.[8, 17, 22]

Energy cost in terms of V_{O_2} (a parameter which is only valid for aerobic activity) is given for walking by the expression

$$V_{O_2} = 1.8 VW(0.073 + x/100),$$

where V is velocity in metres per minute, W is body weight in kg and incline angle is given in terms of x per cent (being 0 for horizontal walking).[8] The basis for this expression is that 1.8 is the oxygen intake in ml per minute for 1 kg m of vertical work.

There do not appear to be reliable figures for the energy cost of race walking, particularly at speeds of $11-16$ k.p.h.

Running There is substantial agreement that the energy cost of running is rectilinearly related to running velocity, at least up to velocities of 400 m/min. There are also surprising indications that mechanical efficiency is maintained at a high level (22.7 per cent) during heavy anaerobic running at 450 m/min.[9] At marathon running speeds (about 300 m/min) there is a metabolic cost of 60 ml O_2/min/kg,[26] i.e. for a 70-kg runner the cost would be $V_{O_2} = 60 \times 70 = 4200$, which lies within the aerobic ranges of top-class marathoners. Further examples of energy costs of various types of running are best obtained from standard references.[2, 4, 17, 22]

Vertical stepping The implications of vertical stepping within sport are not so obvious, other than in hill climbing, hilly cross-country races, and *standing pedalling* during cycle racing. However, this mode of locomotion allows direct calculations in terms of work output (body weight × height raised) – all simple positive work in the case of stairway and moving stairway climbing, but complex positive and negative work in stepping on and off a one or two rise step. The negative work of stepping down is approximately $\frac{1}{3}$ of the positive work of stepping up.[19] Expressions for the total work done in stepping should take account of the work of standing erect and the work of stepping horizontally forwards and backwards in addition to up and downwards[19]

$$Vo_2 = \text{standing } Vo_2 + 1\cdot33 \text{ (horizontal } Vo_2\text{)} \\ + 2\cdot4 \text{ (vertical ascent)}$$

Cycle pedalling   This activity is considered to be fundamentally different from the others in that the body weight does not have to be supported by the performer. Careful consideration will show, however, that a major part of the cyclist's body weight is supported by his arms and trunk musculature, and even occasionally by his legs. The energy expenditure in cycling is directly proportional to the work done, the plot of the linear relationship having a slope of approximately $2\cdot0$.[7, 13, 20]

Energy requirements

In terms of dietary intake there are unfortunately few athletes who assess their competitive energy needs and evaluate the most effective method of ensuring that energy is there when required, and supplemented *before* hypoglycaemia occurs rather than after signs and symptoms have appeared. The problem divides into two facets:

(1) total daily requirements – usual diet;
(2) specific competitive requirements – dietary supplements.

Daily requirements   The precise measurement of a sportsman's daily energy requirements is a difficult, if not impossible, task. The athlete's body weight is perhaps the best of indices since an excess of intake over expenditure will be reflected in body fat increases. An insufficient intake will result in decreased work output or body weight losses. It has been calculated that the basal energy output of a 70-kg man is 2000 cal per day — just lying in bed and eating. Superimposed on that base will be the requirements of that part of the athlete's life which is sedentary, and then also of that part which is training and competition. East Germany has devoted a great deal of research to sport in recent years, and one area of attention has been the daily energy requirement of good class sportsmen.[11] Sports competitions were divided into five types:

(1) sports with a predominantly cyclic course of activity;
(2) sports with a sharply acyclic course of activity;
(3) sports with a pronounced demand on reaction and strength over short periods of time;
(4) sports with running and jumping types of performance;
(5) sports with more or less equal demands for high ability in strength, endurance and reaction.

A similar subdivision has been made in more physiological terms,[26] from the viewpoint of stamina only (see Fig. 3.16, p. 102).

According to the first of the two classifications, most comprehensive surveys were undertaken to derive a table of average daily requirements for a variety of sportsmen (Table 5.2), with the provisos that:

(1) as skill (mechanical efficiency) develops within these activities, the actual energy requirement may decrease, *unless* the total amount of work done increases;
(2) in the case of female competitors approximately 20 per cent less energy is required for any given activity. No doubt the reader will question some of the categories; there is certainly room for discussion. However, the investigations represent a considerable contribution to the solution of specific problems in sports dietetics.

Specific competitive requirements   Some of the implications of energy supply to working muscles were discussed in

TABLE 5.2 Median energy consumption and corresponding daily food requirements (kilocalories)

Selected disciplines 1	Expenditure of energy/kg of body weight/day (kcal) 2	Average body weight (kg) 3	Normative daily net needs based on computed energy requirements (column 2 × column 3) (kcal) 4	Nutritional, physiological, optimal daily gross requirements, with 10 per cent added for consumption (kcal) 5
Group A				
cross-country skiing	82·14	67·5	5550	6105*
crew racing	69·21	80·0	5550	6105
canoe racing	72·72	75·0	5450	5995
swimming	69·87	76·0	5300	5830*
bicycle racing	80·39	68·0	5450	5995
marathon racing	79·07	68·0	5400	5940
average values (men)			5450	5995*

rounded-off norm: 6000 kcal

Also belonging to sports of group A are skiing, Norwegian combination; middle-distance racing; walking; ice racing; modern pentathlon; equine sports, military; and touring (alpine climbing).

Group B				
soccer	72·28	74·0	5350	5885
handball	68·06	75·0	5100	5610
basketball	67·93	75·0	5100	5610
field hockey	69·18	75·0	5200	5720
ice hockey	71·87	68·0	4900	5390
average values (men)			5130	5643

rounded-off norm: 5600 kcal

Also belonging to group B are rugby; water polo; volleyball; tennis; polo; and bicycle polo.

Group C				
canoe slalom	67·16	68·0	4550	5005
shooting	62·71	72·5	4550	5005
table tennis	59·96	74·0	4450	4895
bowling	62·69	75·0	4700	5170
sailing	63·77	74·0	4700	5170
average values (men)			4590	5049

rounded-off norm: 5000 kcal

Also belonging to group C are circuit cycle racing (1000–4000 metres); fencing; ice sailing; and gliding.

Group D				
sprinting	61·77	69·0	4250	4675
running: short to middle distances	65·62	65·0	4250	4675
pole vault	57·83	73·0	4200	4620
diving	69·24	61·0	4200	4620
boxing (middle and welter weight: to 63·5 kg)	67·25	63·0	4250	4675
average values (men)			4230	4653

rounded-off norm: 4600 kcal

Also belonging to group D are hurdle races; broad and high jump; hop skip-and-jump; ballet; swimming; figure skating; figure roller skating; and ski, ski jump, bob sled and tobogganing.

---

* Deviations of a few per cent from the median values are, in the field of biology, to be taken as basically insignificant.

TABLE 5.2—*continued*

Selected disciplines 1	Expenditure of energy/kg of body weight/day (kcal) 2	Average body weight (kg) 3	Normative daily net needs based on computed energy requirements (column 2 × column 3) (kcal) 4	Nutritional, physiological, optimal daily gross requirements, with 10 per cent added for consumption (kcal) 5
Group E				
Group I				
judo (lightweight)	72·92	62·5	4550	5005
weightlifting (light- weight)	69·15	67·5	4650	5115
javelin	56·95	76·0	4350	4785
gymnastics with apparatus	67·14	65·0	4350	4785
steeplechase	63·96	68·0	4350	4785
ski: Alpine competi- tion	71·29	67·5	4800	5280
average values (men)			4508	4959

rounded-off norm: 5000 kcal

Group II				
hammerthrow	62·46	102·0	6350	6985
shot put and discus	62·47	102·0	6350	6985

rounded-off norm: 7000 kcal

Also belonging to group E/I are wrestling; automobile rallies; motor racing; gymnastics; acrobatics; parachute jumping; equine sports, shows; decathlon; and bicycle gymnastics.

Chapter 2. During many forms of competition the body energy stores (whether fat or carbohydrate) are insufficient in magnitude or availability to cope with temporary demands of the event. In such cases the sportsman must have access to supplementary energy; indeed, in some long distance events the regulations prescribe the positioning and function of feeding stations quite precisely.

When energy supplements are required, there are several criteria governing selection and usage: speed of assimilation and transport to working muscles; palatability (taste and consistency); low bulk – high energy yield; and legality.

Glucose has long been favoured as an oral energy supplement for sportsmen. It is assimilated very rapidly, a rise in blood glucose being quite marked within 10–15 minutes of ingestion. It can be the most concentrated oral dietary supplement a sportsman can obtain, and does not offend international doping regulations. There have been some problems in the past with the palatability of glucose, especially as a powder, but now glucose is available in much more appetising forms. Glucose syrup has been very thoroughly investigated [12] under a variety of conditions approximating to many different competitive events. In all cases it proved to be an extremely effective supplement, but needed careful use in order to achieve optimal benefits. Of greatest importance was the ingestion of the syrup at such times as each individual sportsman's glucose assimilation curve could best counter an *anticipated* hypoglycaemia. Waiting for hypoglycaemia and then applying the remedy gave some benefit, but not to the same extent as carefully timed tailor-made schedules.

In some long duration events, regular feeding with glucose syrup (a mixture of mono-, di- and polysaccharides, hydrolysing to dextrose) maintains the blood glucose at higher than normal levels throughout the event. In one trial (of uninterrupted rowing, cycling and treadmill running for 100 hours without break) the only ingestion allowed was of

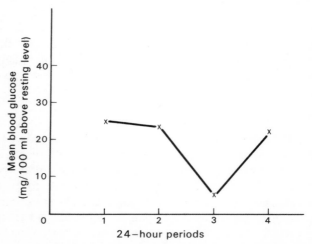

Fig. 5.4 Mean blood glucose levels during 100 hours of continuous exercise (means calculated from 24 readings at hourly intervals)

glucose syrup starting 36 hours before exercise, which maintained a male subject's mean blood glucose 19·2 mg/100 ml
higher than normal throughout (Fig. 5.4).[30]

This trial demonstrates that a true physiological steady
state can be established at low levels of work. The subject
covered the equivalent of 100 miles on the treadmill, and
260 and 170 miles respectively on the cycling and rowing
ergometers. After 48 hours of 'running in', a steady state of
heart rate response was reached which was remarkably free of
diurnal variations. Blood glucose and other physiological
parameters remained relatively steady, while psychological
parameters such as mental recall and vigilance exhibited a
steady and cyclic deterioration. In spite of mental tiredness
therefore, a sportsman can be treated as a metabolic machine
for extremely long periods, being fed sufficient fuel to maintain his energy output at a more or less constant level.
Glucose syrup is probably the most efficient fuel for this
purpose.

Though not as extreme as the previous example, a wide
variety of trials has indicated the supremacy of glucose syrup
as a rapid fuel replacement over the whole range of competitive events.[12] Increased efficiency (in terms of lower heart
rate for standard work loads), increased output (in terms of
greater maximum work loads) and decreased fatigue effects
both during and post competition, are the usual effects of
proper competitive diet.

Metabolic servicing

For the competitor, the second major reason for eating is the
anabolic function of digestion. Replacement of worn body
tissue, and hypertrophy of tissue, are fundamental to the
principles of training. Fuel may be necessary to provide
energy for training, but body building elements are necessary
for the training to have effect. The fat deposit mechanism of
body growth has been discussed previously (p. 145). The building of other body tissues is largely a matter for proteins, vitamins and minerals, with which cells synthesise special structures

and chemical compounds. Through the continuous deamination process of the liver (for energy or excretion) there is a
continual mean loss of protein amounting to at least 45 gm
per day.

The method by which proteins accomplish their function is
described in Chapter 1. However, protein ingestion has long
been a fetish in sports, and it is important to separate fact
from fantasy. The total daily protein demand of the stable
adult sportsman is 1·5 gm/kg body weight, though athletes
undergoing periods of accelerated growth may require far
greater amounts. The ratio of animal proteins to vegetable
proteins should be equal to or greater than 1. The protein
intake should represent approximately 15 per cent of the total
diet. Despite the claims for high protein diets, except in
certain 'gross body' activities it is harmful to exceed an intake
in excess of 2 gm/kg bodyweight. There is a risk of functional
overloading of renal and hepatic dissemination, leading to a
deterioration in metabolism and deficiency of vitamins and
potassium.

Vitamins   The close relationship between vitamins and
physical performance, in terms of enhancing both energy
production and body structuring, is well established. Physical
performance decrements are the first manifestation of
hypovitaminosis. In sports activities there is an increased
demand for vitamins, which may generally be catered for by the
large increase in normal dietary intake. There is considerable
debate over the taking of vitamin supplements in sport. Even
those who support supplementation disagree concerning
quantities and balance. Perhaps the most significant contribution has come from the Austrian physiologist Prokop,[24] who
not only demonstrates the importance of regular supplementation of vitamins C and E, but also that a destruction of the
proportionate balance between some vitamins (particularly A,
B_1, B_2, B_6, C and E) can reduce performance potential. In this
case, balanced supplementation is necessary rather than large
doses of one or other. Prokop also provides a useful table of
average consumption of vitamins (Table 5.3).

TABLE 5.3   *Average vitamin consumption for an athlete weighing 70 KG*

Vitamin	Nonathlete, mg	Speed/strength performances		Endurance performances	
		Training period, mg	Contest period, mg	Training period, mg	Contest period, mg
A	1·5	2	2–3	3	3–6
B₁	1·5	2–4	2–4	3–5	4–8
B₂	2·0	3	3	3–4	3–4
Niacin	20·0	30	30–40	30–40	40
C	70·0	100–140	140–200	140–200	200–400
E	7–10	14–20	24–30	20–30	30–50

Salt–water balance The reasons for sweating and the effects of this and other water losses will be discussed in Chapter 6. At this stage, the absolute and relative amounts of water and salt in the body should be considered since they are both concerned in digestion.

The amount of body fluid has been discussed in Chapter 1. If that amount is suddenly increased by drinking a litre of water, which is rapidly absorbed from the intestine, there is then a slight increase of about 2 per cent in plasma volume. This increase has a negligible effect on normal body functions.

If there is continuous water depletion in the body through prolonged sweating, a sportsman may lose over 2·5 litres in an hour, 9 litres in 5 hours, perhaps 16 litres per day. In the laboratory, sweat losses of 4·2 l per hr have been recorded.[5] Against a total of 50 litres body water, such a loss is a critical factor in performance. Indeed, a loss of 15 litres is considered to be an immediate precursor of death in a clinical situation.

Water loss tends to be accompanied by feelings of thirst, and most competitors are well advised to slake their thirst as and when it occurs. That this mechanism may not be sufficient was demonstrated with football players, who have been observed to lose large volumes of sweat ($\bar{x} = 5$ lb, max = 14 lb) in spite of drinking sufficient water to abolish sensations of thirst.[18] Despite the larger absolute water loss of the larger sportsman, the relative loss of water is greatest in the small athlete, who is therefore at greater risk of dehydration. In situations of great sweat loss, three stages of dehydration have been described (Table 5.4).[1]

TABLE 5.4   *Signs and symptoms of dehydration in man*

At indicated deficits of body water		
1–5 % body weight	6–10 % body weight	11–20 % body weight
thirst	dizziness	delirium
vague discomfort	headache	spasticity
economy of movement	dyspnea	swollen tongue
anorexia	tingling in limbs	inability to swallow
flushed skin	decreased blood volume	deafness
impatience	increased blood concentration	dim vision
sleepiness	absence of salivation	shrivelled skin
increased pulse rate	cyanosis	painful micturition
increased rectal temperature	indistinct speech	numb skin
nausea	inability to walk	anuria

* Items arranged in approximate order of first appearance as dehydration in the heat progresses to exhaustion and beyond.

The sportsman possesses the usual powers of stress acclimatisation in response to sweating. If commonly exposed to heavy work in warm temperatures, he increases his sweat rate to a higher norm. Though this improves his ability to work under such conditions, it also increases his susceptibility to dehydration. Part of the acclimatisation process therefore must involve an increase in the quantities of fluid ingested.

There is apparently no cause for concern over the possibilities of superhydration (ingestion of more water than is being lost). Athletes performing a test to exhaustion have been shown to suffer a decrease in performance when dehydrated, and an *increase* in performance when superhydrated.[5]

Apart from the subtle imbalances at cellular level which result from water depletion (see Chapter 1), the gross limitation on athletic performance seems to arise from the reduction in plasma volume and the increase in blood density, with its attendant implications upon circulatory mechanics (Chapter 3). Fortunately, the plasma's propensity for giving up water during sweating (2·5 times greater than any other body water compartments) is offset by its favoured place as the immediate recipient of water from the intestines.

Salt losses   Sweating causes a simple sodium chloride depletion. There is a uniform decrease in both sodium and chloride ion concentrations in the extracellular fluid, causing osmotic pressure to shift water into the cells, which then swell. The disturbance of sodium ion concentration is sufficient to upset the efficiency of muscle and nerve cell function; indeed, salt deficiency is manifested mainly as a sodium lack.

In heavy work, severe sodium deficiency causes widespread cramps, which may be overcome by direct saline ingestion. The mechanism of cramp was discussed in Chapter 2. Sweat is normally a 0·2 per cent solution of salt, which may on acclimatisation become weaker. Sufficient replacement of salt can be obtained by a calculated intake of salt in solid form, or more reasonably by drinking a fluid equal in salt dilution to sweat. It is extremely important that sweat losses are not merely replaced by water. Salt deprivation does not cause symptoms of thirst and an athlete may satisfy his water thirst without satisfying his less subjectively detected hyposalinity.

Alcohol   The consumption of alcoholic drinks is so much a part of the social pattern within which the majority of athletes live that it is difficult to separate the athlete from the 'temptation' of alcoholic ingestion. In some sports alcohol is absolute anathema, whereas in others (cycling, for instance) it is positively encouraged for some competitors. The majority of writings and pronouncements about alcohol in sport are so clouded by prejudice and taboo as to conceal the major facts. Alcohol certainly has a psychological effect, and could conceivably be used as a psychological tool by sports coaches. In the physiological sense, alcohol must be viewed as a fuel, and as an ergogenic affector or pharmacological agent.

Alcohol is a high calorie content food, providing 7·2 calories per gram. With a fine sense of discrimination, the first extraction of food elements from the digestive tract is indeed of alcohol, which is taken through the stomach walls. High performance sportsmen are unlikely to be suffering from chronic alcoholism, and this text is concerned solely with acute or short-term effects of alcohol.

A correlation exists between blood alcohol concentration and impairment in sensorimotor performance, the relationship between the two being an exponential function.[14] Concentrations in excess of 0·1 per cent in the blood produce measurable deteriorations in many types of physical performance.[6, 14] These effects are not experienced by all athletes — since some individuals apparently are not subject to such performance decrements — and isometric strength and local muscular endurance appear to be unaffected whereas dynamic power, reaction, coordination and posture control are affected.[16, 21] Cardiocirculatory efficiency is also impaired during locomotion.[15]

In summary, it may be stated that:

(1) alcohol is of negligible food value in sports performance;
(2) alcohol has a deleterious physiological effect on almost all sports performance;
(3) alcohol may have a useful psychological effect on a certain few individuals in sport.

Excretion

Excretion can be subdivided into fluid and solid systems, though they are not absolute divisions since solid excreta still contain fluid, and fluid excreta solids.

Fluid excretion

Sweat   We have seen earlier (p. 158) that much fluid can be excreted via the sweat mechanisms. There are two types of sweat gland, eccrine and apocrine. Eccrine are generally distributed about the body surface in the deep dermis, being densest on the palms and soles, next dense on the head, and least dense on the trunk and limbs. Apocrine glands arise from hair follicles, and are found mainly in the axilla and in the labia majoris and mons pubis of the female. Sweating in sport, therefore, is mainly an eccrine gland function, and is increased by the following stimuli:

(1) temperature rise (a) body temperature,
                                  (b) environmental temperature;
(2) emotional stimuli, the effect being limited mainly to the soles and palms;
(3) during exercise, using the mechanisms of (1);
(4) during nausea, fainting, hypoglycaemia.

In addition to sweat, which is a specific response to stimuli, described in Chapter 6, fluid is also lost via a constant and insensible diffusion of water through the skin, amounting to about 500 ml per day, and termed perspiration.

Vapour   A similar amount to that lost through perspiration is also excreted insensibly through the lungs. While at rest, this equals approximately 500 ml per day. This figure may be greatly increased by virtue of any increase in the daily ventilation rate of the sportsman. However, the total increase in water vapour lost is hardly significant in comparison with sweat losses.

Urine   Urine is formed in the kidneys, which act as regulators of the concentrations of most substances composing the extracellular fluid. Figures 5.5 and 5.6 show the macroscopic and microscopic structures of the kidney. The urine-forming unit of the kidney is the nephron (Fig. 5.7), of which there are approximately one million per kidney. The

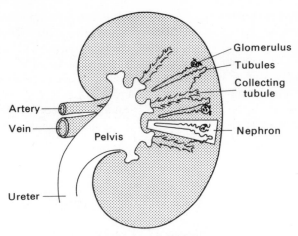

Fig. 5.5 Principal anatomic structures of the kidney

nephron is composed of two basic parts. The glomerulus acts as a filter and removes water and solutes from the blood through its membrane which is extremely permeable to these but not to plasma protein. The glomerular filtrate is therefore virtually deproteinised plasma. This extraction is accomplished by the usual processes of fluid mechanics discussed in Chapter 1. Normally 180 litres per day are processed in this way; thus the total body fluid may be purified several times a day.

The second part is composed of the renal tubules, which reabsorb from the filtrate those elements which the body needs and pass them into the bloodstream. The renal tubes also eliminate those elements unnecessary to the body – such as urine which flows into the renal pelvis and then via the ureter and bladder to be voided by urination. This is the vital process of the kidneys, and functions by either reabsorption or by diffusion and osmosis (see Chapter 1).

Active reabsorption   Glucose, amino acids and proteins, uric acid and sodium, potassium, magnesium, calcium, chloride and bicarbonate ions are reabsorbed by special chemical transport mechanisms. The nutrient absorption mechanism is so powerful that virtually none pass into the urine – *in normal circumstances*. However, electrolyte reabsorption is variable, acting as a control element which is discussed in Chapter 6, particularly of sodium chloride which occupies 75 per cent of the filtration function. Since the active transport system may proceed in opposition to the actual pressure gradients of substances concerned, it is very demanding in terms of

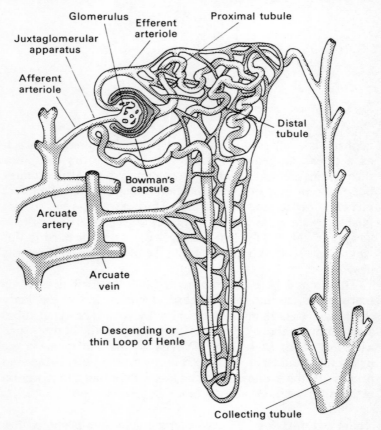

Fig. 5.6 The nephron (modified from Smith, H. W.: *The Kidney*, Oxford University Press, 1951)

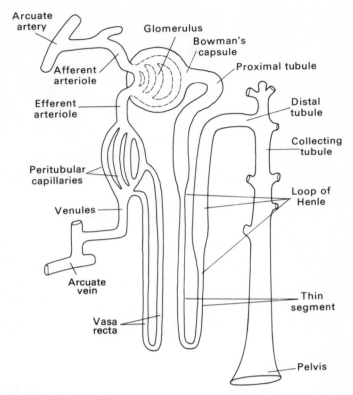

Fig. 5.7 The functional nephron

energy. The tubular epithelial cells require very great amounts of nutrition, in a similar fashion to the requirements of most cellular membranes.

Diffusion and osmosis   Most of the water reabsorption in the kidney occurs by osmosis, which is a reaction following the active transportation of the solutes through the tubules. A large concentration difference is established across the membrane, which therefore causes osmosis of water to redress the balance.

The net result is that all but about one litre of renal fluids per day filter back iinto the bloodstream, the remainder being excreted by urination. The contents of the urine are normally water plus unwanted substances, viz. urea, creatinine, phosphates, sulphates, nitrates, uric acid and phenols. All these substances are waste products of body metabolism, and are potentially harmful if not excreted. Levels (both absolute and relative) of some of these substances may be used to monitor the course of training stress. Particularly, protein urea follows severe exercise — the excretion of proteins may be increased 100-fold,[23] though the athlete decreases this level through training. Some of these proteins may originate from the kidney tissue rather than the plasma.

Additionally, some sportsmen experience a massive rise in urinary sugars which is not pathologic. Such glucosuria is a result of the great increase in plasma glucose which overloads the filtration capacity of the tubules.

Many imbalances discovered in urine composition are relative in view of the decreased urinary output of a sportsman suffering dehydration. It is extremely important for the sportsman to maintain a sufficiently high fluid intake to maintain a normal urinary flow, and allow optimal renal function.

Solids excretion

By the time the chyme reaches the large intestine digestion has virtually ceased. A certain amount of water and perhaps glucose and salt is removed during its passage through the colon. The chyme therefore becomes more solid faeces. The only significant secretion of the colon is mucus, which assists the passage of faeces from the iliocecal valve to the anus. This mucus also protects the intestinal wall from the digestive actions of faecal enzymes. The distal end of the colon is less well protected, and during diarrhea an athlete may experience discomfort from the too rapid arrival of strong enzymes in the distal intestine.

A more common problem of sportsmen is temporary constipation caused psychologically (e.g. by disturbance of routine), or by dietary changes, such as taking iron supplements. In these cases the faeces are longer exposed to intestinal dehydration and become over-solid. A reflex inhibition of defaecation may occur, leading to a vicious circle. The resulting discomfort, if not medically relieved, may inhibit performance considerably.

Experiments in digestive function

Students having access to more sophisticated laboratory facilities, and/or to experimental nonhuman animals, will be best advised by their tutors concerning suitable experimentation. There is still much to be learned from 'black box' studies of the functioning sportsman.

Referring to p. 248 for a reminder of suitable experiment construction, the student is advised that parameters may be divided into certain subgroups. One or more items from each group *may* be examined on one experiment, with *all* groups being investigated or one or more groups held constant during the experiment. Where constancy cannot be ensured, then assumptions about fluctuations may be made by referring to standard tests and their descriptions of such fluctuations. On a within subject basis (test–retest) such assumptions are less critical.

Since digestive effects are less immediate than other body parameters, experiments are in general carried out over much longer time periods, maybe of days and weeks.

Ingestive input:
  (a) calorific value (actual or estimated);
  (b) composition:
      (i) carbohydrate;
      (ii) fats;
      (iii) proteins;
      (iv) vitamins;
      (v) minerals;
      (vi) water;
  (c) timing, absolute and relative to competition;
  (d) bulk and form (fluid, solid, powder, tablet, etc.).

Subjective effect:

    (a) hunger;
    (b) thirst;
    (c) discomfort (of abdomen, mouth, etc.);
    (d) ingestive effort (time and energy of eating, both normal and during exercise).

Physical output:

    (a) energy expenditure (including work modes);
    (b) quality of performance;
    (c) body composition (total mass, relative components);
    (d) excreta (faeces, urine, sweat, breath).

Environment:

    (a) season of year;
    (b) living conditions:
        (i) noise;
        (ii) air conditioning;
        (iii) temperature;
    (c) altitude.

Physiological responses:

    (a) cardiac (rate, acceleration, ECG);
    (b) ventilation (rate, volume);
    (c) blood (glucose, red cell count);
    (d) temperature (surface, core and intra tissue).

References

1. ADOLPHE, E. F. *et al.* (1947) *Physiology of man in the desert.* Interscience Publishers: New York.
2. ASTRAND, P. O. (1952) *Experimental studies of physical working capacity in relation to sex and age.* Munhsgrand: Copenhagen.
3. BALKE, B. (1960) In, *Human biodynamics in medical physics.* Ed. O. H. Glasser, Year Book Medical Publishers: Chicago.
4. BALKE, B. (1963) *A simple field test for the assessment of physical fitness.* CARI Report 63–6, Federal Aviation Agency: Oklahoma.
5. BLYTH, C. S. and BURT, J. J. (1961) 'Effect of water balance on ability

to perform in high ambient temperatures'. *Research Quarterly of the American Association for Health, Physical Education and Recreation*, **32**, 301.

6. CARPENTER, J. A. (1962) 'Effects of alcohol on some psychological processes'. *Quarterly Journal of Studies on Alcohol*, **23**, 274.
7. CHRISTENSEN. H. (1931) 'Die Körpertemperatur während und unmittelbar nach Schwerer Körperlicher Arbeit'. *Arbeitsphysiologie*, **4**, 154.
8. ERICKSON, L. *et al.* (1946) 'The energy cost of horizontal and grade walking on the motor drive treadmill'. *American Journal of Physiology*, **145**, 391.
9. FENN, W. O. (1930) 'Functional and kinetic factors in the work of sprint running'. *Americal Journal of Physiology*, **93**, 433.
10. GOLDBERG, L. (1943) 'Quantitative studies on alcohol tolerance in man'. *Acta physiologica scandinavica*, **51** Supp., 16.
11. GRAFE, H. K. (1964) *Optimale Ernährungsbilanzen für heistungs sportler*. Akademic-Verlag: Berlin.
12. GREEN, L. F. and THOMAS, V. (1971) 'Some effects of glucose syrup ingestion during vigorous exercises of differing intensities and durations'. *Proceedings of the Nutrition Society*, **31**, 5A.
13. GRIMBY, G. *et al.* 'Cardiac output during submaximal and maximal exercise in active middle aged athletes'. *Journal of Applied Physiology*, **21**, 1150.
14. HEBBELINK, M. (1954) *Invloed van Alcohol op het Menselijk Organisme bij Rust en Arbeid*. Licentiate Diss., University of Ghent: Belgium.
15. HEBBELINK, M. (1962) 'The effects of a small dose of ethyl alcohol on certain basic components of human physical performance. I. The effect on cardiac rate during muscular work'. *Archives internationales de pharmacodynamie et de thérapie*, **140**, 61.
16. HEBBELINK, M. (1963) 'The effect of a moderate dose of ethyl alcohol on certain basic components of human physical performance. II. The effect on neuromuscular performances'. *Archives internationales de pharmacodynamie et de thérapie*, **143**, 247.
17. MARGARIA, R. *et al.* (1965) 'Energy cost in running'. *Journal of Applied Physiology*, **18**, 367.
18. MURPHY, R. J. (1963) 'The problem of environmental heat in athletics'. *Ohio State Medical Journal*, **59**, 1.
19. NAGLE, F. J. *et al.* (1965) 'Gradational step tests for assessing work capacity'. *Journal of Applied Physiology*, **20**, 745.
20. NAGLE, F. J. *et al.* (1966) 'Comparison of direct and indirect blood pressure with pressure flow dynamics during exercise'. *Journal of Applied Physiology*, **21**, 317.

21. NELSON, D. O. (1959) 'Effects of ethyl alcohol on the performance of selected gross motor tests'. *Research Quarterly of the American Association for Health, Physical Education and Recreation,* **30**, 312.
22. PASSMORE, R. and DURMIN, J. V. G. A. (1955) 'Human energy expenditure'. *Physiological Reviews,* **35**, 801.
23. POORTMANS, J. and VAN KERCHOVE, E. (1962) 'La protein urie d'effort'. *Clinica Chimica Acta,* **7**, 229.
24. PROKOP, L. (1965) 'Vitamins and sports performance'. *Periodical for Nutritional Research, Supplement,* 4, Steinkopf: Darmstadt.
25. SCHMIDT-NIELSON, K. (1964) *Desert animals: physiological problems of heat and water.* Oxford University Press: New York.
26. THOMAS, V. (1970) *Science and sport.* Faber: London.
27. THOMAS, V. (1971) 'The effects of glucose syrup ingestion on extended locomotor performance'. *British Journal of Sports Medicine,* **5**, 4.
28. THOMAS, V. and HAMLEY, E. J. (1967) 'Physiological and postural factors in the calibration of the bicycle ergometer'. *Journal of Physiology,* **191**, 2.
29. THOMAS, V. and REILLY, T. (1973) *Observations of professional soccer players.* In preparation: Liverpool.
30. THOMAS, V. and REILLY, T. (1973) *Extreme endurance work with glucose syrup as the fuel.* In preparation: Liverpool.

CHAPTER SIX

Control

All human function is subject to control. Philosophical concepts of individual freedom seem to ignore the existence of
physiological controls which maintain our very existence.
Without control we would die.

Sports performance is a matter of control. The athlete
manifests himself through the existence and manipulation of
his own control systems; he 'nurtures his nature' and draws
from his resources that which comprises his athletic achievement.

Certain basic concepts are necessary to the understanding
of physiological control. In a text such as this, a no more than
cursory definition can be given. Advanced students will wish
to refer to standard texts in cybernetics and control theory.
These concepts centre around two main areas – homeostasis,
and the processing of information.

Homeostasis

Although the human can exist in a wide variety of environmental conditions, and can survive rapid and massive changes
in his external environment, his *internal environment* remains

remarkably stable.[4] The term homeostasis was coined to describe this state.[7]

Information processing

Control is effected by the processing of information. Generally, control systems receive information from a variety of sources, collate and compare this information with models of desirable states, compute instructions to achieve model performance, pass instructions to an effector mechanism, monitor the effects of these actions and feed the information back into the system. The whole system may be represented by the control diagram in Fig. 6.1.

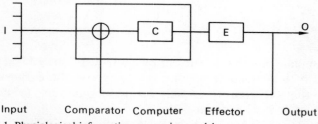

Input   Comparator Computer   Effector   Output

Fig. 6.1 Physiological information processing model

In physiological terms, each of these control system elements has its parallel.

Input Information input may be in many forms, and generally is classified by which of the senses receive the information. The major forms are (a) via the exteroceptors (from the external environment): sound, light, taste/smell, pressure and temperature; and (b) via the interoceptors (from the internal body environment): movement, position, temperature, pressure, acidity and stretch tension.

In those cases where control is achieved by nerves, the information is encoded at the nerve endings into nerve impulses, processed as such, and decoded into whatever nature of output is required by the effector mechanism. In many cases, at least part of the information transmission is chemical, messages being carried via the circulation, and the control system is then neurochemical.

Feedbacks   In most physiological cases, the model effect which the control system is trying to achieve is a constant level of some parameter or other, e.g. body temperature. In control theory the fixed value is termed a set point and the difference between the actual output of the system and its set point is returned as an error message via the feedback loop. This is called negative feedback, and in the case of body temperature, the negative feedback mechanism acts in the same way as a thermostat. However, the body thermostat is far more complex than a motor car thermostat (which operates on *plus* error messages to bring a cooling system into play) or a domestic thermostat (which operates on *minus* error messages to bring a heating system into operation). In fact it combines systems, controlling fluctuations either way, as will be shown later in this chapter. The essential point is that in a negative feedback system error messages cause alterations in effector messages which tend to return the output towards set point. It can now be seen that homeostasis and physiological set point are synonymous.

In some cases, feedback control acts as a positive system. Starting from some point an increase in output feeds back to create *further* output, and so on in a vicious circle which is usually found in pathologic or traumatic sports situations. In a happier sense, positive feedback can be seen in the training overload situation where the more the sportsman improves his fitness, the more he needs to train to improve his fitness still further — and so on.

One important concept to the sportsman is that a physiological set point may be varied. In fact, the process of acclimatisation seeks to accomplish changes in set point which will enable the athlete to function more efficiently in response to increased competitive demands or to changes in the environment. It is this function, for example, which allows marathon runners to perform at core temperatures in excess of clinically extreme ranges.

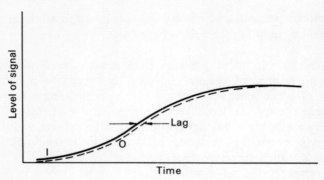

Fig. 6.2

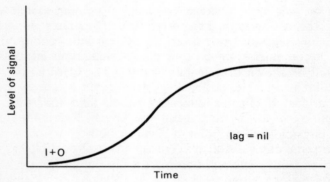

Fig. 6.3

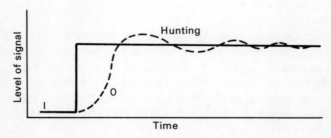

Fig. 6.4

Modes of control   Control signals follow typically different modes to fit the particular demands of any given function.

(i) Direct.
    (a) The monitoring of output gives immediate signals to alter the output. The time consumed between detection of error and the repairing of that error is called lag. The alteration of output is by continuous fluctuation (Fig. 6.2).
    (b) The effector signals are based on a *prediction* of what will be required, and we have predictive control. This tends to eliminate lag but depends upon accurate prediction (Fig. 6.3).

(ii) Hunting. A sudden change in input produces a lag in output. The output then follows input as quickly as it has power to do, and overshoots the desired (set?) point, returns and overshoots and so on in ever decreasing oscillations (Fig. 6.4).

Heart-rate response to exercise provides good examples of (i) and (ii). In (i) (a) a gradual increase in workload will be accompanied by a slightly lagging increase in heart rate. In (i) (b) an anticipatory increase in heart rate might coincide with, or indeed even precede the increase in work load. In (ii) an abrupt change from hard work to resting will be followed by a

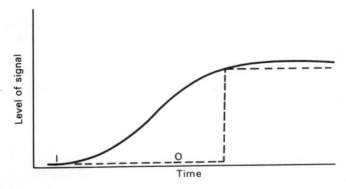

Fig. 6.5

lag in falling heart rate, and then a hunting for a steadily decreasing plateau (set point).

 (iii) Step. A steadily increasing input cannot achieve an effector output until a certain strength of signal has been achieved (Fig. 6.5). The muscle fibre control described on p. 29 is an example of this form of control.
 (iv) Rhythmic. A rhythm of output is maintained in response to a steady input (Fig. 6.6). Peristalsis and heart pacemaker functions are of this type.

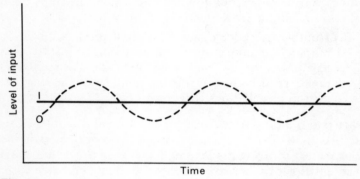

Fig. 6.6

Those who seek to optimise sports performance, that is to control the performance of an athlete, should understand the mechanisms underlying those performance parameters with which they are dealing.

The nervous system

A moment's thought will be sufficient to make one realise that the functioning sportsman is an immensely complex organism, the workings of which are mostly not understood. Even that which is understood is too vast and complex to be fully described in a few thousand words. On the other hand the

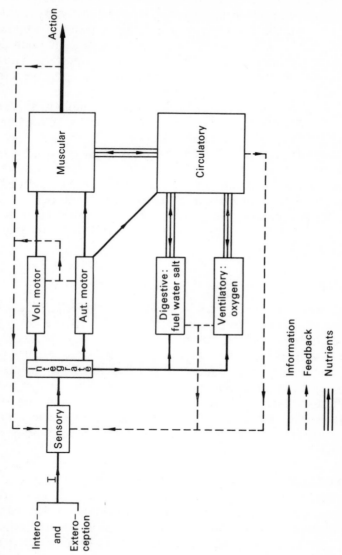

Fig. 6.7 Network of physiological systems

sportsman has to be guided in his training and competition whether by himself or his coach. Even when the most sophisticated of guidance systems such as the East German computer based training schemes are used, their success rests upon the potential for understanding possessed by the sports scientists who construct them. So, however inadequately, sport must try to obtain a general view of and for each sportsman.

The sportsman's control systems are amenable to this approach. Figure 6.7 shows a simple representation of the interlocking of the major systems covered in Chapters 2–5, with the nervous system which achieves most body control for the sportsman. It can be seen that the sensory nervous system deals with the encoding of input information and the transmission of that information to the integrative nervous system (the human computer, in popular parlance). The effector messages are then handled by the autonomic and voluntary motor nervous systems.

The information organs

Information is handled by neurons, or nerve cells. The long filaments growing from the neurons are the nerve fibres or axons, some of which are extremely long since the neurons are located mainly in the brain and spinal cord. Figure 6.8 illustrates a typical neuron. The membrane of the axon actively transports sodium ions out of the fibre and into the interstitial fluid – the sodium pump. Since sodium ions are positive the result of the sodium pump is to create a normal resting membrane electrical potential of about 85 millivolts.

A sudden increase of permeability of the membrane to sodium allows a sudden surge of sodium ions to the inside of the fibre which overshoots the midpoint (see p. 175 for overshoot control), and causes a reversal of the polarisation, called depolarisation. Potassium ions tend to fill the 'vacuum' left by the sodium ions and diffuse out through the membrane, carrying a positive charge and eventually repolarising the nerve. Since the permeability of the membrane to sodium is depen-

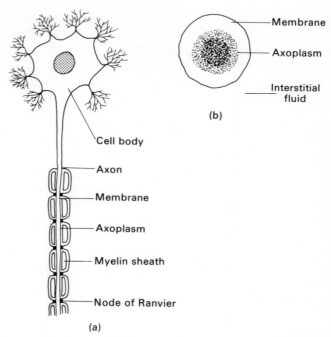

Fig. 6.8 (a) A nerve cell with its threadlike axon, showing the nerve membrane, the axoplasm and the myelin sheath
(b) Cross-section of an axon

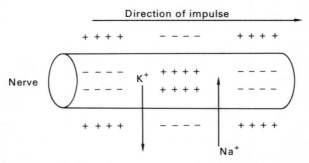

Fig. 6.9 Movements of Na$^+$ and K$^+$ during a propagated action potential (Hodgkin, A. L.: *Biol. Rev.*, **26**, 339, 1951)

dent on the electrical impulse initiating the nerve action, the depolarisation tends to spread along the axon away from the initial stimulus, closely followed (about 0·0003 sec) by the repolarisation. This pulse of electrical change is a nerve impulse and is shown diagrammatically in Fig. 6.9.

Upon depolarisation, the nerve fibre is incapable of being stimulated until after repolarisation has taken place. This is called the refractory period and lasts from 0·0004 to 0·004 sec. Even though the sodium pump may fail to act, the accumulation of sodium inside the cell is so minute at each impulse that very many thousands of impulses can occur before there is a sodium block to further impulses. The free diffusion of potassium across the membrane is sufficient to maintain the repolarisation process.

Nervous stimuli   The excitability of nerve is so great that almost any impulse is capable of acting as a stimulus, though certain special nerve receptors are tuned to certain types of specific stimulus. The more common stimuli are: electrical, chemical, light, sound, pressure, temperature or tension. Different nerves comprising the same nerve trunk have different levels of excitability. As the detected signals become stronger, so the number of nerve fibres stimulated increases; or in control terminology, the larger the amount of information to be transmitted the larger the transmitting medium needs to be.

The speed at which impulses travel along nerves is dependent on two factors.

(i) The presence of a myelin insulating sheath (Fig. 6.8) causes impulses to travel much faster and, incidentally, helps to minimise sodium leak into the fibre. Myelinated fibres tend therefore to be found where fast response is necessary – in rapid body movements and in most sensory situations. Unmyelinated fibres are found in autonomic nerves, and in less urgent sensory nerves such as pain and pressure receptors.

(ii) The larger the nerve, and the thicker its sheath, the faster its impulses move. The largest nerve fibres (about 20 microns diameter) conduct impulses at about 100 m/sec, while the smallest conduct at only 0·5 m/sec.

Nerve fibres can transmit many signals successively at a rate which is limited by their specific refractory period. A period of 0·001 sec for example, would constitute a practical limit of fewer than 1000 impulses per second.

Strength of signal   Nerve bundles utilise the foregoing methods to vary the strength and continuity of their signals. There are therefore two means, operating simultaneously, to accomplish this variation:

(1) Spacial summation, where the required number of nerve fibres all act simultaneously. This method not only allows variation by summation of fibres, but also variation by permutation of fibres of different strength.
(2) Temporal summation, where impulses are transmitted at different rates over the same fibre. Two impulses per second would give a weak signal, whereas 100 impulses per second would be much stronger.

The sensory system

This section of the nervous system (Fig. 6.10) is concerned with the input of the control system. The sensory input is divided into exteroceptive sensation arising from without the body, and interoceptive arising from within the body. Interoceptive sensation is subdivided into proprioceptive (the state of the body – physical tension, pressure, movement, etc.), visceroceptive (the state of the viscera), and chemoreceptive (the chemical levels of the fluids). The input is classified by the level it reaches within the hierarchy of system complexity.

Some signals reach only the spinal cord, crossing the cord to initiate cord reflex actions, which will be discussed later (p. 199). Some signals reach the lower brain, and are more highly organised into motor reactions, though still at a subconscious

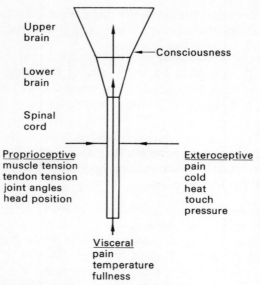

Fig. 6.10 Major information routes of the sensory system

level (p. 201). Yet other signals reach the upper brain (thalamus and beyond), becoming consciously integrated, at the highest level being discretely localised and organised in the brain cortex.

The majority of sensory nerves have free nerve endings, which are relatively nondiscriminating and crude. They may transmit pain, pressure and temperature, and because of their extensive interconnections may confuse one sensation with another. Fine discrimination is achieved by sensory nerves having end organs which are specific to certain categories of stimuli. These end organs may be exteroceptive (sight, sound, fine touch, taste, etc.) or proprioceptive (body position, joint angle, muscle stretch, etc.).

There is also a hierarchy of sensory nerve ability to diminish its receptivity to certain signals. So much information is continually flooding into the nervous system that the sportsman would be in danger of drowning in it. By a process of sensory adaptation, certain types of receptors diminish the strength of signal with continued exposure to a stimulus. For example, the initial shock of entry into a cold swimming pool is gradually dulled; the first touch of the donned football shirt is recorded, but then the sensation of wearing the shirt is quickly lost. Conversely, proprioceptive sensations do not experience adaptation, since the competitor needs to be continually aware of his physical position and state. Other sensations come somewhere between in this hierarchy of adaptation. Pain is one of these, since after the first sharp warning that trauma is present the signals diminish, allowing the sportsman to continue competing while being partially or completely unaware of traumatic pain.

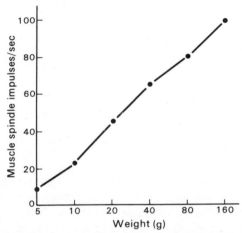

Fig. 6.11 Logarithmic response of the muscle spindle (data from Matthews: *J. Physiol. (Lond.)*, **78**, 1, 1933)

The ability of sensory nerves to discriminate between input signals is a logarithmic function of the intensity (Fig. 6.11).[26] This means that differences between signal strengths are perceived as being relative to the magnitude of the total signal strengths. A basketball player can perceive a difference of 10 gm in a 600 gm ball. A weightlifter cannot perceive a difference of 10 gm in a 10,000 gm weight.

End organs in exercise

The eye

For the competitor, vision is the most important exteroceptive mechanism. Fig. 6.12 shows the basic structure of the eye. The outer layer is a very strong fibrous envelope called the sclera, which is fronted by a clear section, the cornea. The interior of the envelope is filled with the aqueous humour, virtually extracellular fluid, whilst behind the crystalline lens is the vitreous humour, a proteinaceous clear fluid. Between the lens and the cornea is a muscular sphincter called the iris.

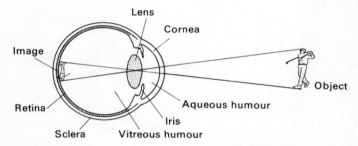

Fig. 6.12 General structure of the eye showing the function of the eye as a camera

Light passes through all these media to strike the retina which contains specialised end organs called rods (which differentiate intensity of light) and cones (which differentiate colours). The retina also contains a layer of very black pigment called melanin which absorbs the light after reception.

The rods greatly outnumber the cones, and are far more light sensitive. In poor light conditions, visual discrimination is achieved mainly by rods, in which case differences in shade are more discernible. In better light, cones can play a larger part, allowing the best differentiation to be by colour. The implications of these phenomena in sports situations are too obvious to need elaboration.

Vitamin A is essential to optic function. Contained in the pigment layer, it combines with proteins in the rods to form rhodopsin. The formation of rhodopsin is a continual process; it is broken down to its constituents by light energy which excites the rods and cones thus initiating the nerve stimulus. The length of a single visual nerve signal is approximately 0·1 sec, irrespective of the duration of visual stimulus. Therefore, when a succession of visual stimuli are presented at a rate in excess of 10 per sec, fusion of signals occurs. This is the underlying principle of moving pictures which generally operate at 16–32 frames per second.

The eye is enormously adaptable to variations in the strength of visual information. Its adaptation is achieved by two coordinating mechanisms:

(1) the iris muscle contracts, thus reducing the aperture, called the pupil, through which light enters the lens;
(2) the sensitivity of the rods and cones changes; since rhodopsin is broken down by light energy, a continued exposure to intense light will gradually deplete the rhodopsin in store, thus reducing sensitivity. Conversely, in very low light levels, the store of rhodopsin increases enormously, thus increasing the sensitivity. This adaptation has a power of varying refined sensitivity by a factor of 100 000. Adaptation to darkness is a relatively slow process, taking about an hour to reach its maximum, whereas light adaptation requires only about ten minutes.

For these reasons, players should be given adequate time for adaptation to whatever playing environment they are to enter, or be allowed a similar environment immediately prior to competition.

Visual acuity describes the clarity of the images transmitted by the eye. It is dependent upon the function of the iris in focusing light rays sharply on to the retina, particularly a small central area of the retina called the fovea which has only specially small diameter cones. Perfect eye focusing is called emmetropia and is measured in terms of an individual's ability to see clearly at a distance of 20 ft what a normal person can see at 20 ft — thus 20 : 20 is normal vision. If he can only see clearly at 20 ft what a normal person can see at 40 ft or 50 ft, his vision is said to be 20 : 40 or 20 : 50. Exceptionally well sighted individuals may have 20 : 16 or 20 : 12 vision.

A lack of visual acuity will be due to a failure of the lens to converge light rays sufficiently on to the retina — termed hypermetropia or farsightedness (objects being clearer at a distance); or an over convergence of rays — called myopia or nearsightedness; or, more seriously, a distortion of the rays which makes accurate focusing impossible at any distance — called astigmatism.

Visual field Though fine focusing is possible only for a limited area in the centre of the total visual image, the remainder of the area is still available for gross perception. In fact, it is extremely important for the sportsman to possess, and indeed to develop the use of, a wide visual field. Each eye is capable of receiving lateral visual stimuli from 90° to its central axis, being prevented by physical structures (nose, eyebrows) from utilising this field in all directions. However, with binocular vision, an athlete can have a lateral visual field of 180°. Because the point at which the optic nerve enters the retina has no rods or cones, there is a blind spot for each eye which is only detectable when using a single eye.

Depth perception In many sports, the ability to estimate distance is of fundamental importance. It is dependent upon two basic methods (Fig. 6.13):

   (1) size of retinal image — which is compared with a learned expectation of the normal size of such images. For example the retinal image of a football at 20 m is larger than the image of one at 40 m. Through learning what different sized retinal images of footballs mean in terms of distance, the player can estimate the distance between himself and the ball;

   (2) parallax — using the slightly different angles at which

the two eyes receive images to determine depth. This can be done by comparing the object with a known reference point (e.g. a player's position relative to the goal), or by purely identifying the angle of convergence of the two eyes.

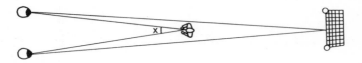

Fig. 6.13 Visual perception of depth

(a) The brain knows how wide a footballer's image is at different distances, (b) the distance represented by $\angle X$ is known, and (c) the distance to the goal is known, and the footballer's position can be compared with that known distance.

The ear

Though some especially dedicated (and occasionally successful) competitors are deaf, most sportsmen rely to a great extent on audible information. A game of squash played wearing efficient ear mufflers will convince students of this fact.

The ear is a structure especially adapted to collect sound energy and transmit it to nerve and organs. Figure 6.14 shows the basic structure of the ear. The external appendage of the ear is a cartilaginous edifice (especially convoluted in boxers and rugby forwards). An aperture in the convolutions leads via the external auditory meatus to the tympanic membrane which is formed of connective tissue covered with skin externally and mucous membrane internally. The membrane is connected to a lever system composed of three bones called ossicles within the inner ear; they are called in order the malleus, incus and stapes. Movements of the tympanic membrane

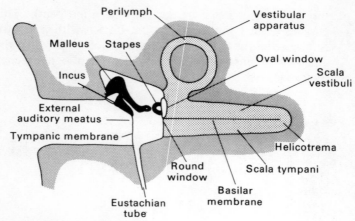

Fig. 6.14 Basic structure of the ear

are thereby transmitted through the inner ear to the oval window of the cochlea, which is a coiled tube filled with lymph. Since air pressures are being transformed into liquid pressures, the lever system is necessary in order to magnify the force and overcome the greater inertia of the liquid. The movements are transmitted through the cochlear lymph to the round windows and detected by the cochlear nerve. The eustachian tube connects the middle ear with the pharynx, passage of air being permitted during swallowing actions, thus allowing the air pressure to equilibrate on either side of the eardrum. Voluntary equilibration is occasionally necessary in subaqua sports and skiing.

Sound travels as waves of pressure. These waves operate over a range of frequencies, the human ear being most sensitive to frequencies between 1000 and 3000 cycles per sec (cps). The maximum frequency capable of detection by the human ear is about 20 000 cps. The pitch of the sound is dependent upon the frequency of the waves. On the other hand the quantity of sound is a function of the amplitude of the waves, and is measured on a decibel scale, which is logarithmic. A scale of typical sound intensities reveals a factor of about 1 billion (English) between the top and bottom.

Decibels	Sound
120	pneumatic drill
100	loud motor horn
80	very heavy traffic
50	conversation, single voice
20	whisper
0	faintest audible noise

At above 120 db, sound can be physically felt, and becomes painful.

Sound discrimination   In especially noisy situations, sportsmen may experience difficulty in perceiving certain important audible signals – the instructions of a basketball coach during play, with a noisy crowd, for example. Discrimination can be improved in two ways:

(1) by giving the signal at a different pitch from the surrounding noise (a referee's whistle, for instance);
(2) by giving a signal of greater volume against a varied noise background (shouting, or a starter's pistol).

Hearing malfunction   Sportsmen may lose the capacity to hear certain parts of the frequency range, or to perceive sounds of low magnitude. In either case, signal systems can be designed to operate within the easily detected range of the individual.

Vestibular apparatus   Situated adjacent to each internal ear is the vestibular apparatus, composed of the utricle and saccule (or the otolith) and the three semicircular canals (Fig. 6.15). The semicircular canals are membranous tubes set in each of three planes at right angles to each other. They are filled with lymph, and open into the utricle which communicates with the saccule via the ductus endolymphaticus. The saccule is then united with the cochlear duct of the ear by the canalis reuniens.

The wall of the utricle contains the macula, which possesses hair-like nerve cells projecting into a jelly called otoconia containing small calcified granules. When the sportsman's head is moved from a central erect position, the weight of the otoconia causes the hairs to fall in that direction, providing the stimulus for nerve messages of proprioception. Additionally, sudden acceleration or deceleration causes the otoconia to lag behind under their own inertia, resulting in proprioceptive signals of loss of balance.

The crista are located at the end of each semicircular canal. They also have fine nerve hairs projecting into the fluid of the

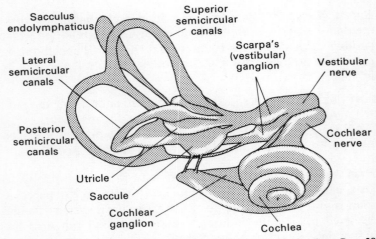

Fig. 6.15 Anatomy of vestibular apparatus (modified from Hardy: *Anat. Rec.*, **59**, 1934)

canals. Sudden changes of direction in any plane cause the fluid within the corresponding canal to flow past the hairs, which bend and transmit the information as a nerve impulse.

The sum total of the vestibular activities, therefore is:

(1) to orientate the head in space, acting as a reference point for orientating the remainder of the body;

(2) to measure accelerations and losses of balance;

(3) to monitor changes of direction.

The importance of these functions is mainly in those sports involving gross body skills. In activities which require particularly complex and rapid body movements (such as diving, gymnastics and dance) the stress is laid upon head position as being fundamental to the performer's proprioception.

The skin

Special end organs in the skin detect information concerning temperature, touch and light pressure. They generally consist of a connective tissue capsule for the demedullated axon, and fall into the following categories important in sport:

(1) Meissner corpuscles, which are rapidly adapting touch detectors. They are normally most prevalent in finger tips, nipples, lips and body orifices;
(2) Pacinian corpuscles, which are quickly adapting pressure detectors most prevalent in the limb extremities and near tendons and joints;
(3) Ruffini organs, which are found generally, and respond to temperature.

The skeleto-muscular end organs

The information emanating from muscles and joints is detected and transmitted by the following end organs:

(1) joint receptors – mainly of three types
   (a) Ruffini organs within the joint capsule are very sensitive to joint *movements*
   (b) Golgi organs – are situated in the joint ligaments and respond to joint *positions*
   (c) Pacinian corpuscles in the ligament are responsive to *acceleration* and quick movements
(2) muscle spindles – are fusiform structures lying parallel to and in between the muscle fibres, which respond to *stretching* of the muscle.
(3) tendon organs – are Golgi organs, and respond to *stretching* in the muscle tendon.

These end organs are responsible for a continuous flow of information about the positions and movements of body segments, and the tension in muscles, which use the vestibular information to build a complete status of the competitor within his environment.

Visceral end organs

These organs are similar to the exteroceptive organs of pain, pressure and temperature. They are situated variously in the viscera and central organs, though they are also receptive to stimuli from deep tissues in the head, muscles and bones. Normally, visceral sensations do not become conscious, but in the event of severe stress or trauma, pain and pressure can be felt – either directly or as referred pain in some other (surface) area. The most important stimulus for visceral pain is ischemia, which probably lies at the root of stitch, and certainly is the root of cardiac pains which are detected in the shoulder region. Other causes of visceral pain are chemical irritation, tissue stretching and visceral muscular spasm.

Chemoreceptors

There are two important chemoreceptors within exercise. The first is the carotid body, a collection of epitheloid cells lying within the bifurcation of the carotid artery. The carotid body really acts both as a chemoreceptor in detecting anoxic anoxia, and as a baroreceptor in responding to the pressure of the pulse wave.

The second are the aortic bodies, found at the root of the right subclavian artery and variously around the aortic arch. Their structure is similar to the carotid bodies, and both sets of chemoreceptors function as a linked unit.

The motor nervous system

The motor nervous system conducts information from the body control centres to the effector mechanisms of the body.

While the sensory system deals with the things experienced by the body, the motor system is concerned with 'doing things'. The motor nervous system is therefore concerned with controlling muscles of all types, and some of the glands. In this case, rather as in the treatment of sensory nerves, the discussion will be limited to the distal end of the nerves. At this site, non-nervous phenomena (energy) are transformed into nerve impulses in the sensory mechanisms, and the reverse occurs in the motor mechanisms.

Skeletal muscular function   The method whereby skeletal muscle fibres are caused to contract by nerve stimulation has been extensively covered in Chapter 2. Voluntary movements of the sportsman, including subconscious coordinations and skills, are catered for by this system. Though there is not a hard and fast division, the remainder of the sportsman's function can be considered within the province of autonomic function.

Autonomic nervous system   This system operates involuntarily to control and maintain many of the internal organic functions of the body. The system divides neatly into two sections on anatomic, hormonal and functional counts; the sympathetic division, which prepares the sportsman for competition, and the parasympathetic division, which stimulates vegatative functions.

Sympathetic nervous system   Figure 6.16 illustrates how the short sympathetic nerves (white rami) arise in the spinal cord, pass out to form a chain on each side of the cord, from which the sympathetic nerves proceed to (a) the viscera or (b) via another small nerve (grey ramus) into the spinal nerve, travelling with it to its ultimate destination.

Parasympathetic nervous system   The majority (90 per cent) of the nerve fibres in this system originate in the 10th cranial

194   Exercise Physiology

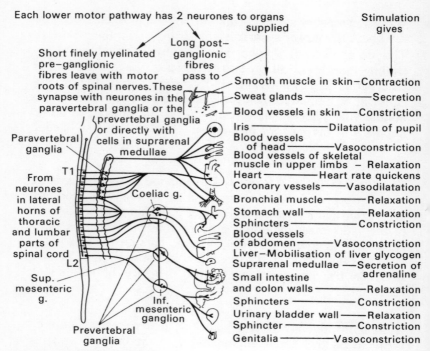

Fig. 6.16 Sympathetic outflow

nerve, the vagus. The remainder originate from the 3rd, 7th
and 9th cranial nerves and from a few of the sacral nerves
(Fig. 6.17).

Nerve junctions

Since information may travel through several nerves between
sensory input and motor output, there must be junctions
between the ends of the nerves. These junctions are termed
synapses (Fig. 6.18).

The axon is that part of the neuron which transmits information from the cell body (or soma). The dendrites, of which
there may be from one to several hundred, transmit information to the cell body. Lying on the surface of the soma and

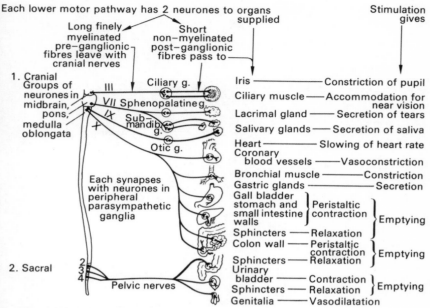

Each lower motor pathway has 2 neurones to organs supplied

Stimulation gives

Long finely myelinated pre–ganglionic fibres leave with cranial nerves

Short non–myelinated post–ganglionic fibres pass to

1. Cranial Groups of neurones in midbrain, pons, medulla oblongata

III   Ciliary g.
VII Sphenopalatine g.
IX   Sub-mandib. g.
      Otic g.

Each synapses with neurones in peripheral parasympathetic ganglia

2. Sacral

2 3 4

Pelvic nerves

Iris —————————— Constriction of pupil
Ciliary muscle ——— Accommodation for near vision
Lacrimal gland ——— Secretion of tears
Salivary glands ——— Secretion of saliva
Heart ———————— Slowing of heart rate
Coronary blood vessels ——— Vasoconstriction
Bronchial muscle ——————— Constriction
Gastric glands ——————— Secretion
Gall bladder stomach and small intestine walls } Peristaltic contraction } Emptying
Sphincters —— Relaxation
Colon wall —— Peristaltic contraction } Emptying
Sphincters —— Relaxation
Urinary bladder ——— Contraction } Emptying
Sphincters —— Relaxation
Genitalia ———— Vasodilatation

Fig. 6.17 Parasympathetic outflow

dendrites are the presynaptic terminals of the axon branches coming from many other neurons. The junction between the terminal and the dendrite is called a synapse.

The transmission of a nerve impulse at the synapse follows the same pattern as the action of the neuromuscular junction explained in Chapter 2, with the important difference that the neuromuscular junction secretion is of acetylcholine which acts as an excitatory chemical of muscle. At autonomic synapses, most sympathetic neurons secrete noradrenaline; the parasympathetic secrete acetylcholine. Additionally, the spacial and temporal summation effects mentioned earlier in this chapter have effect at the synapse, particularly since there is a synaptic threshold of excitation below which the axon will not transmit. Once this threshold has been exceeded, and for so long as the potential remains above the threshold, the axon will fire repetitively at a rate which is proportional to the level

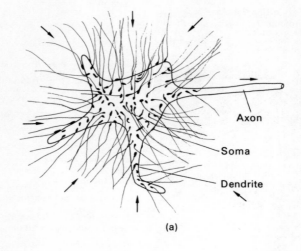

(a)

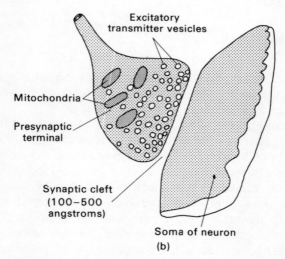

(b)

Fig. 6.18 (a) Typical neuron, showing hundreds of presynaptic terminals that
originate from other neurons
(b) Physiological anatomy of the synapse

of the potential. If the discharge of the postsynaptic terminals is insufficient to cause an axon firing, the potential will gradually accumulate, facilitating the neuron so that a relatively small additional discharge will trigger the axon. In some nervous sportsmen, a large number of neurons can become facilitated without actually firing. A very small additional stimulus can then cause a sudden and disproportionately large response. Some athletic events of an explosive nature are very amenable to this build up approach in locomotor nerves.

Unlike nerve fibre transmission, synaptic transmissions are extremely liable to fatigue – some more so than others. This fatigue allows nervous actions to die away gradually, or make way for other signals. A huge repetition of impulses passing through a synapse gradually achieves a permanent facilitation of the synapse. Similar impulses are facilitated through the system, making the repetition of motor performance more efficient. This is one of the mechanisms used in the training of a sportsman, particularly in repetitive skills.

The integrative nervous system

This section of the nervous system deals with descriptive information received from sensory nerves, and gives instructional information to motor nerves. It functions through a hierarchy of levels ranging from the absolutely simple to the infinitely complex, the complexity generally correlating with the level of the system to which the information rises.

The anatomy of the system can be seen in Fig. 6.19.
In this system three major levels of integrative function can be delineated:

(1) spinal cord – concerned mainly with basic reflex action
(2) brain stem – concerned mainly with subconscious function
(3) cerebral cortex – concerned with thinking and voluntary discrete motor activities.

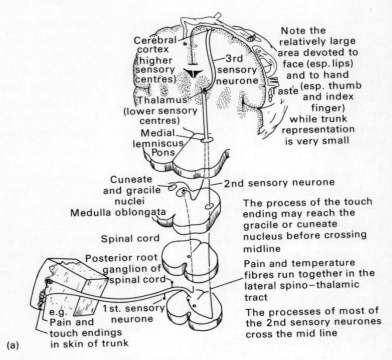

Note the relatively large area devoted to face (esp. lips) and to hand (esp. thumb and index finger) while trunk representation is very small

The process of the touch ending may reach the gracile or cuneate nucleus before crossing midline

Pain and temperature fibres run together in the lateral spino–thalamic tract

The processes of most of the 2nd sensory neurones cross the mid line

Fig. 6.19 (a) Sensory pathways and cortex

The nerve endings registering pain, warmth or cold, touch and pressure are linked by a chain of 3 neurones with final receiving centres in the sensory area of the parietal lobes. The exact points to which impulses come from different regions are indicated

Spinal cord

The spinal cord is situated within the central column of the spine and is formed of ascending and descending tracts, describing long nerve fibres which carry information upwards or downwards; cell bodies of cord neurons which form the grey matter; and propriospinal fibres which connect one region of the cord with another (Fig. 6.20). The reflex actions of the spinal cord take the path shown in Fig. 6.21. The spinal cord reflexes normally elicited in sport are shown in Table 6.1.

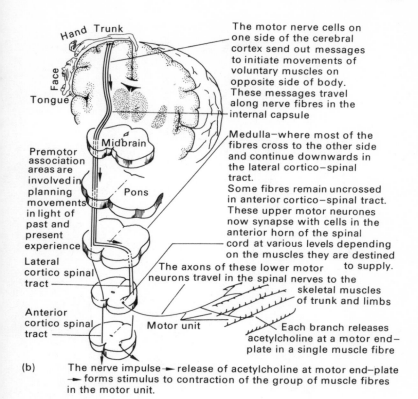

(b)   The nerve impulse→ release of acetylcholine at motor end–plate
→ forms stimulus to contraction of the group of muscle fibres
in the motor unit.

Fig. 6.19 (b) Motor pathways to trunk and limbs
The controlling centres in the motor cortex are linked by 2 neurones
with the effector organs – the voluntary muscles

During competition, the sportsman is continually utilising
these reflex actions to perform much of his function. The fact
that the information integration occurs at the level of the
spinal cord assists him in that he does not occupy any of his
valuable higher integrative centres in performing reflex skills
(particular conscious integration), and the shorter route taken
by the nerve impulses means they take effect in a shorter
time.

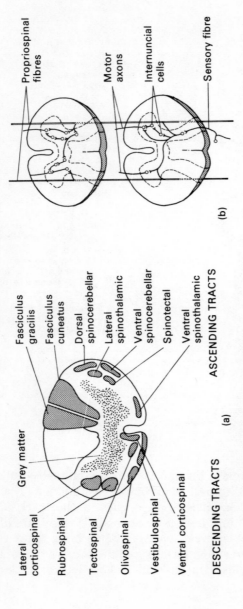

Fig. 6.20 (a) Fibre tracts and grey matter of the spinal cord
(b) Two segments of the cord, illustrating the internuncial mechanisms that integrate cord reflexes and the propriospinal fibres that interconnect the cord segments

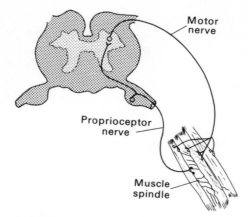

Fig. 6.21 A typical spinal reflex arc – the stretch reflex

TABLE 6.1 *Spinal cord reflexes*

Description	Stimulus	Receptor	Synapse	Action
Stretch reflex	sudden muscle stretch	muscle spindle	single	contraction of agonist
Tendon reflex	excessive tendon stretch	tendon Golgi	multiple	relaxation of agonist
Extensor thrust	pressure on pad of foot	Pacinian cell	internuncial	contraction of extensors
Flexor reflex	pain	pain end organ	internuncial	flexor withdrawal
Crossed extensor	pain	pain end organ	internuncial	extension of opposite limb
Reciprocal inhibition	excitation of a muscle	any	internuncial	relaxation of antagonists
Locomotor	locomotion	several	internuncial	rhythmic function of locomotor muscles

Brain stem

The brain stem itself divides into two parts (Fig. 6.22):

    (a) The lower brain stem – the medulla and the pons; and
    (b) the mid-brain – mesencephalon.

Their function can be seen as both motor and autonomic. The

motor functions are concerned mainly with dynamic and static posture in the sense of achieving equilibrium and of opposing the attempts of gravity to destroy that equilibrium. Earlier in this chapter, the vestibular apparatus was described. The vestibular information is carried to the vestibular nuclei within the lower brain, where crude integration is performed and motor impulses transmitted. This postural integration is performed in the presence of a great amount of information from other sources, sensory from the body, and proprioceptive and motor from the upper brain.

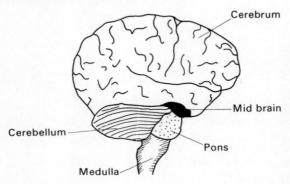

Fig. 6.22 Parts of the brain

The autonomic functions of the brain stem which are of direct use to the sportsman are

(1) respiratory centre, in the medulla;
(2) cardiac centre in the pons;
(3) sympathetic and parasympathetic centres in the hypothalamus;
(4) temperature centre, in the hypothalamus;
(5) water balance centre, in the hypothalamus.

The hypothalamus is particularly important as a centre for establishing the basic state of the body. When stimulated, it can regulate almost all autonomic functions, some directly by nerve impulses and some indirectly through hormonal secretions. Its situation is somewhat marginal, between the mid-

and upper-brain, and it may be described as part of either, certainly in terms of function.

Upper brain

The upper brain is formed of the cerebellum and the cerebrum (Fig. 6.23). The cerebellum is concerned with fine coordination and balance. The cerebrum can be subdivided into (a) the

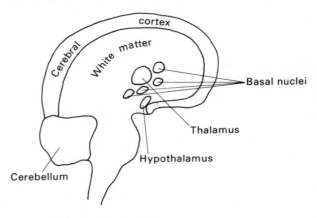

Fig. 6.23 The cerebrum and the cerebellum

cerebral cortex – the outer layer (grey matter) which contains the nerve cell bodies, and constitutes the highest level of nervous function – mental behaviour, thought, consciousness, will, intellect, speech, etc.; (b) the inner (white) matter, which is composed of nerve fibres; (c) basal nuclei, small groupings of grey matter within the white matter; (d) the thalamus, concerned with sensory reception and selection of that which will be relayed to the cortex, and of regulation of highest sensation and movement; and (e) the hypothalamus (see above).

The basal nuclei are closely connected with the cortex and thalamus. They control many of the habitual movement patterns of sportsmen – movements which are more complex than postural movements, but do not require the complex voluntary control which will be used in what are called 'open sports skills'. The cerebellum functions as an overriding buffer or damping mechanism on the other motor controlling areas, reducing the dimensions of control errors and imposing predictive control of some movements (see p. 175). The cortex divides into sensory, motor and integrative areas.

Nervous control of motor functions

When considering this aspect of the athlete's function it is difficult to separate neurophysiology from skills psychology. The area of psychology is seen more clearly when examining motivation, temperament, intelligence, etc. even though these may in part be physiologically based. It is oversimple to merely define psychology as the study of the psyche, and physiology the study of physical body function – the two are inextricably linked.

In this text, it is the physiological basis of sports function which is being studied, and each major subdivision of function will now be examined from the point of view of nervous control. These functions are

spinal reflexes
postural reflexes
involuntary movement patterns } musculo-skeletal function
voluntary movements

cardiac
ventilatory
visceral } autonomic function
thermal

Spinal reflexes

Basic coverage of these functions was given on p. 199. One or two special implications should be mentioned here. The first concerns the stretch reflex. Anatomically speaking, muscles have to be stretched in order to reach from their origin to insertion, which ensures that the muscle spindle constantly maintains an impulse discharge, causing the reflex contraction of the muscle. This may be viewed as a state of readiness of the muscle, called muscle tone. The degree of muscle tone is modified, however, by supraspinal mechanisms, both voluntary and involuntary.[23]

The stretch reflex is also used in emergency situations, where a body segment may be unexpectedly displaced by an external force. The stretching of muscles which occurs reflexly causes them to contract, thus tending to oppose the displacement. This phenomenon is most frequently observed in physical contact games.

Tendon reflexes are extremely important in the prevention of sports injuries. The highly developed and motivated competitor is frequently capable of exerting sufficient muscular force to cause a stretching or even a tearing of the muscular tendon. These ruptures tend to occur to the Achilles, patellar, rectus and biceps (long head) tendons, in running and jumping for the first three, and in throwing and heaving activities for the last. Such ruptures are a result of motivation overcoming the normal tendon reflex.

The extensor thrust reflex is a useful addition to the coordinated control activity of landing on the feet from a height. Most competitors will land on the balls of the feet first, requiring an immediate and powerful extensor activity to absorb the force of landing. Since sportsmen do not generally look at the floor when landing, the extensor reflex is capable of initiating the absorbing extension before the athlete is consciously aware that the feet have contacted the ground.

Reciprocal inhibition (or reciprocal innervation) of antagonists reflexly accompanies all reflex agonist action, and also voluntary movement. It facilitates agonist function by reducing tonic opposition of the antagonist muscles. It can be seen that reciprocal inhibition acts in a contrary manner to the stretch reflex — which of the two gains ascendency depends upon the nature of the stretching movement (whether or not it is effector agonist action).

Postural reflexes

It helps to evaluate sports movement if it is realised that movements start from one posture and end in another, and that while the body is moving either the whole body or parts of it may be exhibiting one or more postures. In fact positional reflexes might be a better term in sports analysis.

Posture is dependent on the degree and distribution of muscle contraction, and is adjusted by neck reflexes, vestibular and righting reflexes. Also of course voluntary cortical activity can modify posture. The discussion might proceed to the consideration of those reflexes which are acquired or modified by habitual patterns of activity – the conditioned reflex. Some postural reflexes in sport are conditioned reflexes.

A rigid physiological definition of a reflex would be, 'responses to peripheral nervous stimuli occurring involuntarily and involving the central nervous system, which are inborn and generally present in normal humans'. However, Pavlov [28] extended the concepts of reflex action to include the subsequent reorganisation of reflexes into new activity patterns. He considered the conditioning process to be basically a cortical activity, and that conditioned reflexes were always built on inborn reflex patterns. Prolonged physical exercise can produce postural adjustments accompanied by sustained alterations in the spinal motor neuron characteristics. [35] Accordingly, many postural conditioned reflexes in the sportsman can truly be called reflex activity, since they are established from basic reflexes, conditioned through voluntary training of the sportsman, and then function involuntarily during sports performance. On a simple level, the hyperextension of gymnasts' and divers' ankles as the feet leave the floor provides a good example of a conditioned postural reflex.

Involuntary movement patterns

The muscular activity of a sportsman is controlled by an overlapping coordination of many different reflexes. [31] Supraspinal control of reflex activities are essential for sports performance. Descending pathways from the brain stem and cerebrum modulate afferent fibres.[9, 23] The lengthy training of the sportsman appears to cause an increase in efficiency of reflex patterns,[3] to some extent by a decrease in the integration delay caused at the synapse.[25, 37]

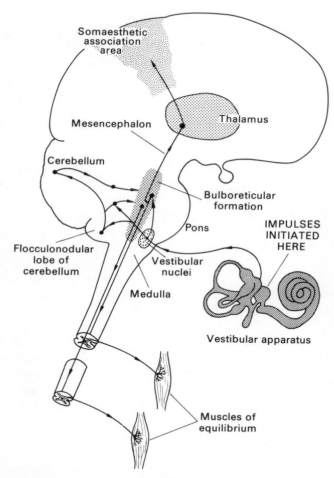

Fig. 6.24 Nervous mechanisms of equilibrium

The coordination of involuntary motor patterns is mainly achieved in the bulboreticular formation of the brain stem, including some of its connections with nearby neural sectors (Fig. 6.24). Information flows into the formation from all body parts via the spinal cord (sensory), from the cerebellum (proprioceptive), vestibular apparatus (equilibrium), and motor cortex and basal ganglia (motor). A widespread stimulus in the upper formation provokes mainly stimulation of the extensor pathways, and is therefore vital to the maintenance of posture against gravitational effects. The relaxation of these stimuli is achieved by inhibitory signals from the basal ganglia. Another important function of the basal ganglia is to coordinate the action of muscles and their antagonists – to damp or control oscillations which otherwise would occur (tremor). This is achieved by a short feedback loop from the bulboreticular formation to the basal ganglia and back.

In sport, the major involuntary movement pattern is locomotion – walking, running, swimming, skating, cycling, etc. Repetitive training achieves a control system which operates (e.g. in the case of walking) in the following way. Spinal reflexes and the bulboreticular formation maintain extensor postural muscle activity, modified by corrective muscular contractions triggered by equilibrium apparatus. From this balanced posture, rhythmic propulsive and balancing movements of the limbs are voluntarily initiated, then becoming involuntary under the control of rhythmic circuits in the spinal cord, with reciprocal innervation circuits maintaining efficient and balanced operation of antagonists. Sudden changes still precipitate vestibular modifying signals, and voluntary alterations of rate and direction merely cause temporary disturbances in the essentially involuntary spinal reflex action.

Voluntary movements

It is unlikely that any examples can be found in sport of completely voluntary movements: the guidelines are as usual somewhat arbitrary. Within this section, it is difficult to establish the borderline for basal ganglia and cerebellar functions. The basal ganglia operate subconsciously, controlling involuntary movements, but also help to control voluntary gross muscle function, gross locomotor patterns, and basic body positioning preparatory to performance of fine motor function. The cerebellum has a most complex function which is especially vital in sports performance. It is a central receiving store of all available sensory information concerning body position and movement, as is also given information about the motor signals being sent to musculature (i.e. information from the cortex about the movements *it is about to perform*). It is therefore the major movement feedback mechanism, sampling its feedback information at several stages in the control process. The more important functions of the cerebellum, therefore, are (a) damping of overshoot; (b) predictive control; and (c) equilibrium.

An overall view of the control of sports voluntary movement can be obtained on a temporal basis. Sensory information reaches the brain and brain stem. Part of the information becomes conscious in the sensory cortex. The integrative cortex decides what action to take, refers to memories of previous actions and instructs the motor cortex to proceed with the action, also referring this action to the cerebellum. The motor cortex sends motor impulses to the musculature, reinforced or modified by feedback signals at all levels of the nervous system. The possible number of bits of information which *could* enter the cortex during this operation is huge. The control system consists therefore of a number of filters, the strength of the filters depending upon both nature and nurture (heredity and training). The sportsman who is concerned with complex function – particularly team games – develops filter systems which relegate as much of his performance as possible to conditioned reflex level. He also lays in a large store of movement patterns from which he can readily select, and develops an efficient search and selection system for these patterns based upon a training in recognition of critical cues in his sensory information array.

Cardiac control

Cardiac muscle fibre is inherently rhythmic in action, having the property of self discharging every time its membrane potential builds up. A group of fibres from the right atrium, called the sino-atrial node (s-a node), have a rate of about once in 0·8 sec, faster than other cardiac fibres. The spread of excitation from the node dominates the somewhat slower rates of the remaining cardiac fibres, so that the inherent cardiac rate is 72 per min, established by the s-a node (sometimes called the pacemaker). This function is no part of the nervous system, but is an essential part of cardiac control. Normal cardiac muscle fibres would be capable of transmitting the pacemaker's impulse throughout the heart, but in order to obtain a more concerted effort in each ventricle, a special group of muscle fibres called Purkinje fibres transmit the impulse six times as rapidly in those chambers. The Purkinje fibres detect the sino-atrial impulse at the atrio-ventricular node (a-v node), situated in the lower part of the right atrium (Fig. 6.25). The sequence of events now becomes:

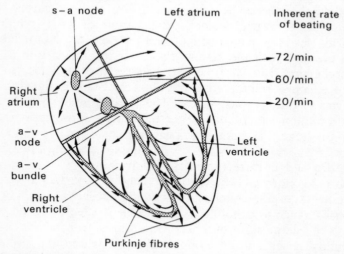

Fig. 6.25 Spread of nervous excitation of the cardiac muscle, and inherent heart rates of different parts of the heart

(1) s-a node originates impulse;
(2) impulse reaches a-v node a few hundredths of a second later;
(3) a-v node delays impulse another few hundredths of a second;
(4) Purkinje transmission takes another couple of hundredths of a second.

This delay ensures that the atria are given time to eject their contents into the ventricles, and the almost simultaneous contraction of ventricular fibres ensures an efficient emptying of the ventricles against arterial pressure.

Superimposed upon this inherent cardiac self control is a system of nervous control (Fig. 6.26) which emanates from the autonomic system. The parasympathetic input is via the vagus nerve, which directly inhibits the s-a and a-v nodes. Vagal tone therefore results in a reduced heart rate, a reduced

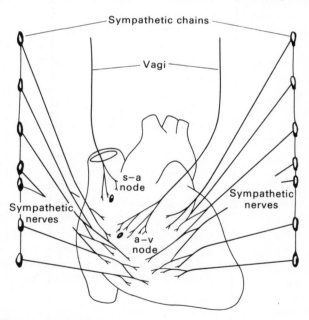

Fig. 6.26 Innervation of the heart

atrial contractile force, a slower a-v node conduction rate, and a decreased coronary circulation.

Conversely, sympathetic stimulation of the heart achieves the reverse effects, increasing the activity of the heart as a blood pump. Sympathetic cardiac stimulation is limited by the normal cardiac fibre refractory period of 0.3 seconds − giving a theoretical maximum heart rate of $60/0.3 = 200$ beats per minute. The observation of exercise heart rates in excess of this figure indicates that sympathetic stimulation may also reduce the cardiac refractory period to perhaps 0.2 sec.

The control of the heart by autonomic means originates from the hypothalamus, but is mediated by many other factors. At this stage it is helpful to take an overall view of the different controls of the heart:

(1) emotional stimulation of the hypothalamus causes both sympathetic and parasympathetic effects;

(2) ventilation phases affect vagal tone which in turn affects heart rate (sinus arrhythmia), both by a leakage of impulses from the ventilatory centre to the cardiac centre and by excitation of vagal stretch receptors in the lung which reflexly increase vagal tonic impulses;

(3) Marey's reflex, in which mean blood-pressure levels are detected by the cardiovascular baroreceptor afferents during resting conditions, and inversely affect heart rate via vagal tone;

(4) Bainbridge 'reflex'; from an initially slow heart rate, a rise in venous return is accompanied by a rise in heart rate. It is not yet certain if this is a reflex in the true sense, and its *modus operandi* is uncertain;

(5) oxygen lack accelerates the heart, which may be due to the action of chemoreceptors (p. 172) but is also possibly due to direct effects on the s-a node;

(6) temperature rises affect both the s-a node directly, and the cardio-acceleratory centre of the hypothalamus via the thermoregulatory centre;

(7) adrenaline directly accelerates the heart rate, whereas noradrenaline increases vagal deceleration via its effect

on blood pressure, detected by the carotid and aortic sinuses;

(8) increases in blood carbon dioxide act directly on the medulla to increase heart rate.

The circulatory responses to exercise were discussed in full within Chapter 3, particularly the heart-rate responses to exercise. It was also demonstrated that cardiac ejection pressures varied. The increase in myocardial contraction force is due to:

(1) greater distension of the cardiac fibres by the larger venous return, which causes a stretch reflex contraction within those fibres;

(2) sympathetic nervous stimulation increases the contractile force in addition to heart rate.

Ventilatory control

Unlike cardiac control, ventilatory control is normally achievable voluntarily. The sportsman *can* control his own depth and rate of breathing consciously, but for the great majority of the time breathing is under involuntary control, even during stressful competition. In Chapter 4, the muscular function of ventilation was described, showing that the active work of ventilation was mainly performed during inspiration, with expiration due mainly to elastic tissue recoil and gravitational effects. The nervous discharge to the ventilatory muscles tends therefore to be a rhythmic inspiratory stimulus, initiated from the respiratory centre in the brain stem.

The motor ventilatory nerves act generally through normal spinal pathways to the muscles concerned, with the exception of the major ventilatory muscle — the diaphragm. This is served by a special nerve, the phrenic nerve. The control of the ventilatory impulses in the sportsman is a complex one. During normal, medium and low intensity activity, the rhythmic function of the respiratory centre may be enhanced by the following sensory inputs:

(1) the basic rhythm is reinforced by the Hering–Breuer reflex, arising from stretch receptors in the lungs. As

the lungs extend, inspiration is inhibited and exhalation enhanced;

(2) the Hering–Breuer reflex also acts as an inhibitory mechanism against over inflation;

(3) carbon dioxide levels in the blood positively affect depth and rate of ventilation, by (a) direct action of carbon dioxide on the ventilatory neurons, thus increasing their excitability and (b) changes in the carbonic acid level in the cerebrospinal fluid (via the blood) which directly influence the respiratory centre (N.B. This negative feedback mechanism is the only control of body carbon dioxide levels.);

(4) body fluid activity – hydrogen ion concentration – directly affects ventilatory neurons in a negative feedback circuit;

(5) oxygen deficiency *can* affect the respiratory centre, via the aortic and carotid chemoreceptors. Since blood oxygen levels very rarely suffer a great decrease, this control system is less common in sport than might be imagined – except perhaps during exertion at altitude where blood oxygen levels may decrease;

(6) arterial baroreceptors feed the respiratory centre, causing negative feedback between blood pressure and ventilation;

(7) Emotional states can cause cerebral cortical stimulation of the respiratory centre;

(8) conditioned responses can be developed which synchronise ventilatory patterns with other functions: (a) with speech; (b) with air availability, e.g. prone swimming strokes; (c) with locomotor patterns, e.g. one inspiration per two running strides; and (d) explosive breathing, e.g. karate, shot putting.

Together, these systems might cause increases in alveolar ventilation in the order of two-fold for oxygen lack, five-fold for acid balance and ten-fold for carbon dioxide excess. However, these feedback systems are so sensitive, and have such short control lags, that oxygen, carbon dioxide and H^+ imbalance is relatively slight, even at very high work loads. It is probable that predictive control is being exercised during strenuous competition by:

(1) simultaneous autonomic stimulation of the respiratory centre by the cerebral cortex along with stimulation of the locomotor musculature system;
(2) sensory information from working muscles flowing partly into the respiratory centre causing reflex inspiratory excitation.

In the sportsman, then, a very high ventilatory level may be maintained in spite of a minimal change in oxygen, carbon dioxide and H^+ levels.

Visceral control

Of major concern to the sportsman is the control of the digestive tract, the major element of which is intramural nerve plexus which is present in the gut wall from the oesophagus to the anus. The plexus controls the gut musculature, and also much of the glandular secretion into the gut.

The intramural plexus receives, mainly via the vagus, parasympathetic fibres which stimulate gut function. Sympathetic fibres from the spinal cord have an inhibitory effect on gut function.

The peristaltic action of the gut is triggered as a stretch reflex, when there is substance within the gut causing the walls to distend. The distension causes a gut contraction on the upper, and a relaxation on the downward, side of the substance, allowing the contents to move downward through the system.

The secretory functions of the gut may be subdivided as shown in Table 6.2. From the sportsman's point of view, the control of gut function is mainly an inhibitory one — sympathetic information causing a suspension of gut function during competition. It is probable that even this reflex control can be conditioned by training, allowing digestion to proceed during training and competition, which is of special importance during long duration events.[36]

TABLE 6.2   *Secretory functions of the gut*

Location	Secretion	Organ	Stimulus
Cell	mucus	mucous cells mucous glands	continual
Mouth	saliva	salivary glands	psychic, and presence of food, via salivatory nuclei in brain stem
Stomach	hydrochloric acid	gastric glands	psychic and presence of food, via medulla
	pepsin		presence of food – local reflex; hormonal, via gastrin
Small intestine	amylase trypsin lipase sodium bicarbonate	pancreas	hormonal (pancreozymin and secretin) some vagal stimulation – but of little importance
Small intestine	bile	liver (stored in gall bladder)	continuous production in liver, release from storage under hormonal control (cholecysto-kinin) and local nerve reflex opening of sphincter of Oddi
Small intestine	sucrase, maltase, lactase, peptidases and lipases	epithelial cells	local nerve reflexes; hormonal system decides *which* secretions are necessary (enterocrinin)
Large intestine	none		

Thermal control

Whereas at rest, the total heat production of the body may emanate mainly from liver, heart, brain and endocrine glands, with only a 40 per cent contribution from the musculature, at severe levels of exercise the muscular contribution may rise to 95 per cent of the total.

Though the rise in body temperature acts as a catalyst of metabolic activity, and a new set point may exist during high levels of exercise, the major part of the heat produced must be lost from the body during extended exercise. If the exercise involves the athlete transferring energy into some other energy-absorbing system (e.g. an ergometer), then some of his potential heat production will be lost in this way. The excess body heat is lost by the physical processes of evaporation, conduction and radiation.

The nervous control of heat loss is by the evaporative mechanism. A small amount of fluid is constantly diffusing through the skin, and the process of evaporating this fluid requires about 0·5 Calorie per gm. The evaporation of insensible perspiration could therefore cater for all body heat lost under basal conditions if perspiration were at a rate of 150 ml per hour. During sports activities evaporation is the critical mechanism for losing large quantities of body heat. Consequently, large volumes of sweat are produced by the sweat glands; the evaporation of this sweat from the skin allows body heat to dissipate.

The production of sweat is closely related to the average temperature throughout the body, or in other words, to the heat per unit mass of the body. The internal temperature is proportional to the metabolic rate. The controls for these functions are mainly nervous. The thermal centre of the hypothalamus responds to increases in blood temperature by reciprocally reversing the activity of autonomic heat production and conservation mechanisms (vasoconstriction, hypermetabolism, shivering), by stimulating the sweat glands via the sympathetic fibres, and by dilating the peripheral blood vessels to allow heat to be carried to the body surface.

The sportsman is rarely concerned with the conservation of body heat during competition, but, if it is necessary, his peripheral vascularity will constrict by reflex inhibition of the sympathetic fibres, the hypothalamus will initiate tonic impulses to the musculature which set up the oscillating contractions called shivering, and there will be a sympathetic increase in metabolic rate.

Autonomic nervous system

The four sections on cardiac, ventilatory, visceral and thermal control have covered the major portion of autonomic function in sport. The overall effect is of course a completely integrated one, and this is summarised by Figs 6.16 and 6.17 and Table 6.3.

TABLE 6.3   *Summary of the autonomic effects of the two systems shown in Figs 6.16 and 6.17.*

Organ	Sympathetic effect	Parasympathetic effect
Eyes (pupils)	dilated	contracted
Sweat glands	increased sweating	none
Gut (glands)	vasoconstriction	increased secretion
Cardiac muscle	increased activity	decreased activity
Coronary blood vessels	dilated	constricted
Abdominal circulation	constricted	none
Muscular circulation	dilated	none
Bronchii	dilated	constricted
Gut walls	decreased peristalsis and tone	increased peristalsis and tone
Gut sphincters	increased tone	decreased tone
Liver	glucose released	none
Kidney	decreased output	none
Basal metabolism	increased	none
Adrenal cortex	increased secretion	none

Hormonal control

The emphasis in this chapter has hitherto been upon control of the functions of the sportsman by the nerves, though in some cases this control has been linked to the release of locally acting hormones – particularly acetylcholine and the digestive hormones. The more important group of hormones are those which are released by endocrine glands for general effect throughout the body.

The regulatory functions of hormones directly affecting sports performance are:

(1) anterior pituitary gland secretes hormones to regulate growth, thyroid hormone secretion and adrenocortical hormone secretion by the adrenal gland;

(2) The thyroid gland controls metabolic rate via the hormone thyroxine;

(3) adrenal medullary hormones have effects similar to those of the sympathetic nervous system;

(4) adrenocortical hormone regulates sodium balance in the kidneys, and partially regulates nutrient metabolism;

(5) pancreatic secretion of insulin regulates glucose utilisation;

(6) parathyroid glands regulate calcium concentration in body fluids.

Anterior pituitary

The anterior pituitary gland is situated close to the hypothalamus. Its secretions are controlled partly by the hypothalamus and partly by feedback response to the blood-levels of its own hormones. It produces three major hormones relevant to sports performance. (a) Somatotrophin (growth hormone) acts independently of other hormones directly on body tissues to stimulate their growth, particularly causing retention of N, P, Ca^{2+}, K^+ and Na^+. It can increase the mass of skeletal muscle (being accompanied by the urinary excretion of creatinine). Its effects in promoting protein synthesis from amino acids, and increased rate of cell division, require the presence of insulin. Somatotrophin is therefore protein-anabolic with high insulin levels. (b) Corticotrophin acts as a general regulator and stimulator of the adrenal cortex – the function of which will be discussed later. (c) Thyrotrophin acts as a general regulator and stimulator of the thyroid.

Thyroid

The thyroid gland has a remarkable capacity to take up iodine from the blood, the iodine pump being stimulated by thyrotrophin. The iodine is used to manufacture two hormones, thyroxine and triiodothyronine, which profoundly stimulate oxidation in almost all body tissues. Thyroxine forms 90 per

cent of the output, and it acts as a feedback to the hypothalamus in controlling the release of thyrotrophin. Its
oxidative effect fundamentally controls body metabolism, and
it also is essential for normal activity of the nervous system.
Thyroxine enhances the intestinal absorption of glucose and
the peripheral glucose utilisation, enhances general glycogenolysis and promotes glucose synthesis from non-carbo-
hydrate sources.

Adrenal medulla

The adrenal gland is composed of two distinct organs – the
medulla and the cortex. The adrenal medulla secretes into the
bloodstream adrenaline and noradrenalin, both of which have
a general effect similar to the sympathetic branch of the
autonomic nervous system. This function is nervously
stimulated by fibres from the splanchnic nerves, which are in
turn stimulated by the medulla and hypothalamus. These
signals may be modified by sensory information from the
sinus and aortic nerves. Adrenaline is the more effective of the
two secretions, except for the effect of noradrenaline in raising blood pressure.

Adrenal cortex

The cortex is, like the medulla, responsive to stress in the
sportsman. It is an essential organ and its secretion of cortisol
(hydrocortisone), corticosterone and aldosterone regulates the
metabolism of nutrients, water and electrolytes. It differs from
the medulla in having no nerve supply, and is therefore controlled by the secretion of adrenocorticotrophic hormone
(ACTH) from the anterior pituitary, which is itself controlled
by the hypothalamus and by feedback of the levels of blood
cortisol and corticosterone. The anterior pituitary does not
control the release of aldosterone, which is a direct response
to sodium and potassium levels in the blood.

Pancreas

The endocrine function of the pancreas (as distinct from its epocrine functions in digestion) is to secrete glucagon and insulin. Glucagon has a sympathetic stimulatory effect on liver glycogenolysis, and may be triggered by decreased blood glucose levels, or by somatotrophin. However, the role of glucagon is thought to be a minor one.

The major role is played by insulin, which increases the withdrawal of glucose from the body fluids in three ways:

(1) it increases storage of glycogen (e.g. in liver and muscles);
(2) it increases the rate of oxygenation of glucose to carbon dioxide in the tissues;
(3) it increases conversion and storage of fats from glucose, and prevents the lipolysis of fat already present in storage.

It decreases the rate of addition of glucose to the body fluids in two ways:

(1) it decreases glucose formation from amino acids;
(2) it depresses conversion of liver glycogen into glucose.

It can be seen that the pancreatic control of carbohydrate metabolism is vital to athletic performance. The release of insulin from the pancreas is a continuous process, the rate of which is mainly controlled by the level of blood glucose, though vagal efferents may parasympathetically increase the insulin outflow.

The insulin presence in body fluids is normally balanced by the inhibitory effects of other hormones – adrenaline, thyroid hormones, glucagon and most importantly somatotrophin. Thus, the ratio of insulin : pituitary hormone seems to control carbohydrate metabolism. A decrease in that ratio, either by lack of insulin or by increase in pituitary action, causes symptoms of diabetes.

A sportsman who is diabetic may expect the development of hypoglycaemia if he is exposed to extremely strenuous or prolonged activity. Carbohydrate supplements are essential in such cases. If the common activity pattern of the diabetic is a strenuous one, then an alteration in his insulin dosages is required. Some diabetic competitors have reached the highest levels of performance, and careful studies have revealed no significant differences in the ability of young diabetics to undertake strenuous training programmes by comparison with nondiabetics.[22]

Parathyroid

The secretion of the parathyroid hormone acts directly to remove calcium from bones, thus raising plasma calcium levels, and increases phosphate excretion from the kidney. The effect is to maintain the calcium ion level in plasma and extracellular fluids within narrow limits. The control of this system seems to be by a direct stimulation of the gland by the plasma calcium levels.

Rhythmic control

The combination of nervous and hormonal control establishes a most complex and comprehensive system, capable of maintaining the homeostasis of the sportsman. However, it is the nature of humans to undertake basic functions in a rhythmic fashion – sleeping, working, ingesting, excreting. The control systems have evolved on a predictive control basis, therefore, so that physiological functions tend to fluctuate rhythmically in anticipation of the fluctuating demands on the system.

There is a strong body of opinion that such rhythms are rooted in a basic 24-hour rhythm inherent in the cells of all animals,[15] and called diurnal rhythms. Many body systems, both nervous and non-nervous depend upon such rhythms and their integration.[14] These effects may be felt not only in negative functions, but in complex voluntary motor actions.[21] Many studies of patterns of rhythmic autonomic behaviour have been investigated, pointing to the existence of what might be called an oscillating set point for all body functions. That this is based on a 24-hour, or 2 × 12-hour, period seems clear,[20, 30] but it has been demonstrated that artificial days (of 21 or 27 hours) can establish a new periodicity in human diurnal rhythms within a matter of days.[2, 24] Complete shifts of phasing can also be accomplished, such as the jet lag suffered by international travellers, or the shift worker's adaptation to a new work time. These adjustments of rhythm generally take about six days to accomplish.[2]

In an oscillating control mechanism, there are peaks and troughs. It is subjectively clear that sports performance is enhanced when occuring at physiological peak periods. The carefully controlled experimentation necessary to prove this phenomenon over a wide range of sports activities has not yet been performed. However, the evidence for retraining of rhythms demonstrates that individual sportsmen can alter their periods of peak efficiency to coincide with the normally expected periods of sports performance. Within the one training establishment, it would be physiologically unsound to have coinciding daily regimes for a footballer who performs mostly on Saturday afternoons, and a basketballer whose games mostly take place during late evening. The implications of these phenomena are discussed in Chapter 7, within the context of acclimatisation.

Control of drugs

The Council of Europe defined doping as the administration of a pharmacological agent which improved performance, accompanied by a concept of moral unfairness and artificiality.[8]

In a text of this nature there is no place for ethical discussion. The effects and control that drugs can have on sporting performance are discussed in the light of available knowledge. Much controversy, and a certain laxity of scientific methodology, has attended this issue. For that reason, this text will seek to take a conservative view, and not venture into areas of doubtful hypothesis. The specialist student of drugs in sport will no doubt seek further sources.

In a field as vast as this, it is essential to categorise, and the first categorisation will be by organic systems. These are the circulatory, digestive, muscular, nervous and respiratory systems.

Circulatory systems   Sympathetic effects are obtained from epinephrine, adrenaline, caffeine, amphetamines, marijuana, psychedelics and catecholamines — they may therefore enhance sports performance in many types of event. Parasympathetic effects may be desired in certain cases of very nervous sportsmen, in which case tranquillisers are effective.

Digestion   Much conflicting evidence exists in this area, which is caused by the failure of many workers to allow for the emotional and social effects of drug taking within their experiments. In fact, with all other experimental variables held constant, the social environment becomes the dominant factor in the digestion of drugs.[27]

Muscular system   Strength of muscular contraction can be increased slightly by caffeine, but in general it can be affirmed that direct strengthening of athletic muscular contraction by drugs has not been proven. Endurance of muscles has been shown in several studies to be unaffected by drugs[10, 11, 13, 18] though the *perception* of exhaustion may be altered in some cases.[6] In some cases male hormones, especially testosterone, increase muscular resistance to acute and chronic fatigue.[5]

Nervous system   The major effects of drugs are to increase or decrease the activity of nerve centres and impulse conduction pathways. The amphetamines have a powerful stimulant effect on the cerebral cortex, and a general sympathetic autonomic effect. Some workers have demonstrated improved physical and sports performance using the drug[1, 17, 34] whereas others have not succeeded in demonstrating the same results.[13, 18] There seems to be general agreement concerning the effects of the drug on the nervous system itself, *but not of an actual improvement in physical performance arising from this effect.*

Cocaine has been shown in even small doses to have a direct sympathetic effect which is accompanied by improved physical performance and recovery therefrom. It is also a dangerous habit-forming drug.[19]

Caffeine has been generally shown to stimulate the cerebral cortex in small doses, and the brain stem and cord in large doses. Its effects are widespread, enhancing almost all nervous function.

Respiration   There is no strong body of evidence that drugs can improve respiratory function in the healthy sportsman. Individual competitors suffering from respiratory defects will utilise medically prescribed drugs of a great variety in aiding their competitive performance.

A general view of those motor functions used by the sportsman leads to a realisation that changes in performance are generally more psychically than pharmacogenically induced. Additionally, performance increments may be obtained more easily and in a greater degree by competitive preparation not involving drugs (Table 6.4).

Growth hormone   In view of current practice in the administration of anabolic steroids, some discussion of their effects ought to be given.

There are two main hormone groups of possible use to enhance growth in sportsmen. The first is pituitary growth hormone, which at this time is of academic interest only, since it is not widely available or used. Synthetic androgen hormones can have great anabolic effects if administered to young sportsmen.

Since steroids are banned in athletic competition and have considerable 'supposed' unhappy side effects, it is difficult to obtain scientific evidence concerning their use by high-class sportsmen. There is some evidence that athletes using anabolic steroids have shown immense increases in body mass and

TABLE 6.4   *Effects of drugs on performance*

Body function	Drug	Effect	Improvement
Accuracy	cocaine	increased cortical awareness	+
Balance	alcohol	body sway increased	−
	depressants	body sway increased	−
	amphetamine	body sway decreased	+
Skill learning	alcohol	decreased acquisition	−
	strychnine	increased learning	+
	caffeine	quicker learning, longer retention	+
Coordination	alcohol	decreased	−
Fatigue	testosterone	increase resistance to muscle fatigue	+
	corticoid hormones	increased recovery	+
	oxygen	increased recovery	+
	sodium bicarbonate	decreased lactate	+
	adenosine triphosphate	increased resistance to fatigue	+
	sodium and potassium salts	increased recovery	+
	glucose	increased resistance and recovery	+
	caffeine	increased recovery	+
	depressants	increased awareness of fatigue	−
	amphetamine	uncertain	?
Reflexes	strychnine	faster reflexes	+
Speed	amphetamine	increased locomotor speed	+

power [29]. The increases are apparently due to an increased protein anabolism which accompanies vigorous training routines and increased protein ingestion. In young men steroid intakes of varying intensities have not been accompanied by physical and performance improvements.[12, 32] In older men there is evidence that the use of methyltestosterone does increase performance, without unwelcome side effects.[16, 33]

Amphetamine function   The function in sport of amphetamine has received more attention than that of any other drug. If taken in doses of 10–20 milligrams, it has a direct effect on the hypothalamic centres, causing anorexia. In its circulation around the body, its effect is to stimulate local secretions of noradrenaline. Its effect, therefore, is virtually an increased conscious or unconscious sympathetic tone.

Experiments in control

This has been the largest chapter. The systems described in it are largely inaccessible to the student of sports performance. Even for the most sophisticated of physiologists, the difficulties of standardisation and access to parameters have led to many a false trail. Even with those parameters which are accessible, performance changes are of such small magnitude as to make their detection and the recognition of their significance within large variance situations difficult. Some parameters, for instance speed of limb movement, may be better measured by increasing the number of repetitions of the movement. A small change of milliseconds per repetition, detectable only with electronic timers, becomes measurable with a stopwatch if a hundred repetitions are performed.

Referring to p. 248 for a reminder of suitable experiment construction, the student is advised that parameters may be divided into certain subgroups. One or more items from each group *may* be examined on one experiment, with *all* groups being investigated or one or more groups held constant during the experiment. Where constancy cannot be ensured, then assumptions about fluctuations may be made by referring to standard tests, and their descriptions of such fluctuations. On a within subject basis (test–retest) such assumptions are less critical.

Input information:

    (a) visual
    (b) aural
    (c) tactile   } exteroception;
    (d) pressure
    (e) heat
    (f) movement (direction and rate)
    (g) acceleration (positive and negative)
    (h) position (posture)
    (i) location (relative to other references) } interoception.
    (j) temperature
    (k) pressure
    (l) stretch

Output information:

    (a) movement;
    (b) sound;
    (c) heat;
    (d) work done.

Integrative performance:

    (a) time elapsed;
    (b) accuracy achieved (motor, intellectual);
    (c) attention;
    (d) coordinative performance.

Control modes:

    (a) direct;
    (b) predictive;
    (c) hunting;
    (d) step;
    (e) rhythmic.

Environment:

    (a) ambience;
    (b) psychological state;
    (c) personality factors;
    (d) social;
    (e) stress (physiological and psychological);
    (f) health.

Nature of control media:
(a) nerve impulses;
(b) chemical ingestion;
(c) heat.

References

1. ALLES, G. A. and FEIGEN, G. A. (1942) 'The influence of benzedrine on work decrement and patellar reflex'. *American Journal of Physiology*, **136**, 392.
2. ASCHOFF, J. (1965) 'Circadian rhythms in man'. *Science*, **148**, 1427.
3. BASMAJIAN, J. V. (1962) *Muscles alive*. Williams and Wilkins: Baltimore.
4. BERNARD, C. (1949) *Introduction to the study of experimental medicine* (English translation). Olmsted: New York.
5. BUGARD, P. (1960) *La fatigue; physiologie, psychologie, et medicine sociale*. Masson et Cie: Paris.
6. BUGAS, Z. *et al.* (1962) 'Effects of stimulant and depressive drugs on physical persistance'. *Psychological Abstracts*, **37**, 261.
7. CANNON, C. (1932) *Wisdom of the body*. New York.
8. Conseil des Europe (1964) *Doping des athletes*. Strasbourg.
9. ELDRED, E. and BUCHWALD, J. (1967) 'Central nervous system-motor mechanisms'. *Annual Review of Physiology*, **29**, 573.
10. FOLTZ, E. E. *et al.* (1943) 'The influence of amphetamine (benzedrine) sulphate and caffeine on the performance of rapidly exhausting work on untrained subjects'. *Journal of Laboratory and Clinical Medicine*, **28**, 601.
11. FOLTZ, E. E. *et al.* (1943) 'The influence of amphetamine (benzedrine) sulphate, d-deoxyephedrine hydrochloride (pervitin), and caffeine upon work output and recovery when rapidly exhausting work is done by trained subjects'. *Journal of Laboratory and Clinical Medicine*, **28**, 603.
12. FOWLER, W. M. *et al.* (1965) 'Effect of an anabolic steroid on physical performance of young men'. *Journal of Applied Physiology*, **20**, 1038.
13. GOLDING, L. A. and BARNARD, J. R. (1963) 'The effect of d-amphetamine sulphate on physical performance'. *Journal of Sports Medicine and Physical Fitness*, **3**, 221.
14. GOODY, W. (1958) 'Time and the nervous system'. *Lancet*, **1**, 1139.
15. HARKER, J. E. (1958) 'Diurnal rhythm in the animal kingdom'. *Biological Reviews*, **33**, 1.

16. HETTINGER, T. (1961) *Physiology of strength*. Charles. C. Thomas: Springfield, Ill.

17. IKAI, M. and STEINHAUS, A. H. (1961) 'Some factors modifying the expression of human strength'. *Journal of Applied Physiology*, **16**, 157.

18. KARPOVICH, P. V. (1959) 'Effect of amphetamine sulphate on athletic performance'. *Journal of the American Medical Association*, **170**, 558.

19. KARPOVICH, P. V. (1965) *Physiology of muscular activity*. W. B. Saunders: Philadelphia.

20. KLEITMAN, N. (1963) *Sleep and Wakefulness*. University of Chicago Press.

21. LASHLEY, K. S. (1951) 'The problem of serial order in behaviour'. In, *Cerebral mechanisms in behaviour*, John Wiley and Sons: New York.

22. LARSSON, Y. *et al.* (1964) 'Functional adaptation to rigorous training and exercise in diabetic and nondiabetic adolescents'. *Journal of Applied Physiology*, **19**, 629.

23. LAURSEN, A. M. (1967) 'Higher functions of the central nervous system'. *Annual Review of Physiology*, **29**, 543.

24. LOBBAN, M. C. (1960) 'The entrainment of circadian rhythms in man'. Cold Spring Harbour *Symposia on Quantitative Biology*, **25**, 325.

25. MARGARIA, R. *et al.* (1958) 'Effect of stress on lower motor neuron activity'. *Experimental Medicine and Surgery*, **16**, 166.

26. MATTHEWS, H. (1933) Drawn from data contained in *Journal of Physiology*, **78**, 1.

27. MOORE, K. E. *et al.* (1965) 'Effects of *d*-amphetamine on blood glucose and tissue glycogen levels on isolated and aggregated mice'. *Biochemical Pharmacology*, **14**, 197.

28. PAVLOV, I. P. (1927) *Conditioned reflexes*. G. V. Anrep (transl.). London.

29. PICKERING, R. J. (1968) 'Those body building drugs'. *Coaching Review*, June 4.

30. RICHTER, C. P. (1965) *Biological clocks in medicine and psychiatry*. Charles C. Thomas: Springfield, Ill.

31. RUCH, T. C. *et al.* (1966) Neurophysiology. W. B. Saunders: Philadelphia.

32. SAMUELS, L. T. *et al.* (1942) 'Influence of methyltestosterone on muscular and creatine metabolism in normal young men'. *Journal of Clinical Endocrinology and Metabolism*, **2**, 649.

33. SIMONSON, E. *et al.* (1944) 'Effect of methyltestosterone treatment of muscular performance and the central nervous system of older men'. *Journal of Clinical Endocrinology and Metabolism*, **4**, 528.

34. SMITH, G. M. and BEECHER, H. K. (1959) 'Amphetamine sulphate and athletic performance'. *Journal of the American Medical Association*, **170**, 542.

35. TOKIZANE, T. and SHIMAZU, H. (1964) *Functional differentiation of human skeletal muscle*. Charles C. Thomas: Springfield, Ill.

36. THOMAS, V. (1971) 'The effects of glucose syrup ingestion on extended locomotor performance'. *British Journal of Sports Medicine*, **5**, 4.

37. TIPTON, C. M. and KARPOVICH, (1966) 'Exercise and the patellar reflex'. *Journal of Applied Physiology*, **21**, 15.

CHAPTER SEVEN

Adaptation

The evolution of the human has been a process of adaptation. 'The survival of the fittest' is a general expression, not merely a sporting one. However, the human adapts not only from one generation to the next in response to the stresses of his environment, but also within his own lifetime to stresses of all kinds. The human who lives a sporting or physically active life adapts to the special stresses which such a life imposes upon him. The process of stressing the sportsman, and his adaptation to these stresses, is called sports training, and it is the means whereby sports performance is improved.

Stress

The realisation of a concept of stress is of relatively recent origin, and the classic formulation published by Selye in 1956 was, 'the state manifested by a specific syndrome which consists of all the nonspecifically induced changes within a biologic system'.[28] A part of the theory constituted a definition of three stages of stress, which are applicable to sports performance. These three stages are part of a general adaptation syndrome (GAS), and are characterised by a consecutive experience of:

(1) alarm reaction to stress;
(2) resistance to stress;
(3) exhaustion by stress.

In previous chapters it has become apparent that in the case of the healthy competitor, and excluding violent trauma, the exhaustion is virtually always reversible. In exercise terms, GAS stage 1 would represent light exercise, stage 2 would involve hard and intensive exercise schedules, whereas stage 3 would involve physical performance to levels of complete collapse (true exhaustion). The adaptation effect is positively related to the level of stress: indeed, lower levels of alarm stage will produce no adaptation in a sportsman, whereas superfit sportsmen may require to function within exhaustion levels to obtain any further adaptation. It is important to realise that a training stress can be applied to *any* function of the sportsman.

More recently, doubts have been cast on the advisability of *overtraining*, or of experiencing extreme stress in the adaptation programme. Cureton has expanded Selye's theory in order to fit it to the competitive situation.[8] He describes five stages of exercise stress:

(1) alarm (marked sympathetic excitement);
(2) resistance (adjustment to the stress);
(3) trained haemodynamics (holding the trained state without harm);
(4) overtraining (temporary exhaustion, but not death);
(5) death (seldom seen).

Without there being a great deal of controlled evidence in support of the concept, this author obtained many impressions from internationally respected sports scientists at the Olympic Congress of 1972 that overtraining could, and indeed did, occur in first-class sportsmen. Fashions in training are similar to *haute couture*. Light training was the vogue in the early part of this century − gradually increasing to the fanatical devotion and masochism of the past two decades. It would be expected that there should now be a swing against overtraining. It remains to be seen if there is a real systematic basis for the theory. What is certain is that the various levels of stress to which the athlete is subjected should be carefully graduated, and planned to reach optimal levels at specific times.

Physiological adaptation

Athletes in training for physiological development (excluding psycho-motor skill training) are mainly concerned with the stressing and adaptation of muscles, including cardiac and ventilatory muscles. In the chapter on control systems it became apparent that the major adaptive developments would occur in the integrative nervous system, which falls into the province of a psychological rather than a physiological text.

Recent advances in research techniques, particularly that of muscle biopsy, have allowed sports scientists to lift the lid off the black box – the human muscle working. Competitive preparation is beginning to include techniques such as alternate starvation and glucose gluttony routines to supercharge muscle glycogen stores, and even storing an athlete's red blood cells for later reinjection to increase his aerobic capacity! Whereas the first is merely an extreme form of natural preparation, the second is an artificial achievement of a natural phenomenon.

Training of muscle in sportsmen has concentrated historically on three areas, muscle strength, muscle endurance and muscle bulk and form (body building) for skeletal muscle only. The last of these is really a form of strength training involving selective hypertrophy among the skeletal muscles. In Chapter 2 the relation between strength and endurance of muscles was described. At this stage a more hypothetical analysis may be made of the adaptation of muscle tissue. The discussion is hypothetical not in the sense that the effects have only been demonstrated in the laboratory, but that they have not been widely demonstrated to have occured in the adaptation of the sportsman. At present it can merely be said that certain facts concerning muscle reaction to training are emerging, which point in certain directions. It is unwise not to scrutinise these facts.

Muscular adaptation

Training leads to an increase in the number and size of mitochondria,[11, 19] and in a change in proportionate content of protein.[15] It also leads to a shift towards fat utilisation in preference to carbohydrate especially as exercise intensity increases (Fig. 7.1). In harness with this shift, there is an adaptation of the lipolytic system in adipose tissue. Training increases the rate of fatty acid release from adipose tissue.[16]

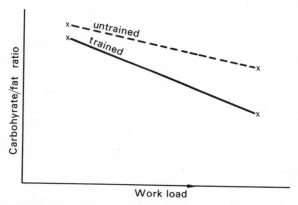

Fig. 7.1 Differences in carbohydrate/fat utilisation with training

These increases in mitochondrial state and components do not seem to play a large part in the achievement of higher levels of Vo_2 max in sportsmen, but rather assist the economy of submaximal work by enabling a greater proportion of muscle to take part in oxidative processes during endurance activities. That is to say, the muscle becomes more 'red'.[5] Since most of the research has been performed on non-human animals, the training processes have been what a human would consider endurance training. It is not surprising that endurance training enhances endurance components of muscular function.

Acute exercise to exhaustion has significant effects on both skeletal and cardiac musculature. There is a gross swelling of some mitochondria, accompanied by a degeneration and disorientation of the mitochondrial christae.[12] It is a recognised technique in body building to 'inflate' the muscles prior to competition with a short bout of severe exercise. This would be compatible with a general swelling of the mitochondria.

The changes in basic structure of mitochondria and christae are transient. Within an 18-hour period the muscle tissue returns to normal.[12] In the sense that the regeneration of exercise breakdown tissue provides an opportunity for hypertrophic effects, this may be the fundamental process of muscle development, associated with an enhanced protein uptake.

A summary of these structural changes[17] suggests that acute heavy exercise results mainly in hypertrophic effects, whilst long duration training produces mitochondrial proliferation. The latter also increases red muscle proportions, and it is possible that heavy power training increases white muscle proportions. Additionally, endurance training increases the resting stores of glycogen in muscle, the usage and amount of fats stored in muscle, the respiratory enzymes in muscle and the total muscle oxygen uptake.[21]

Cardiac adaptation

While cardiac musculature exhibits many of the adaptations to training noted in the previous paragraphs, there are some specific adaptations which are of importance. Throughout the various levels of cardiac function, training increases the vagal tone, which mediates the structural-functional aspects of the heart itself.

Most noticeable, there is a considerable cardiac hypertrophy and chamber dilation (see Chapter 3). Cardiac capillarisation and coronary capacity are increased. Acceleration of heart-rate response to exercise is increased, and deceleration after exercise is quicker. Maximum heart rate may increase, heart rate proportional to set work loads is lower, and basal heart rate decreases. Adaptations to hard training routines create a greater range of systolic pressures and a general lowering of mean blood pressure. There is a reduction in cardiac output at rest and at set work loads, and an increase in maximum cardiac output. The work of the heart is reduced at all levels of activity, and it is capable of reaching higher levels of work output. The daily work of the heart decreases as a result of increased cardiac efficiency.

General tissue

As a general rule well-vascularised body tissues will experience hypertrophy or cell proliferation in response to healthy stress. Increased mineralisation and diameter of bones is commonly reported both during adolescence and adulthood, though the bones of growing children should not be subjected to extra heavy loads. Connective tissues thicken and strengthen with repeated but non-traumatic stress. The tendons of sportsmen, particularly Achilles tendons, are thicker and stronger than in non-sportsmen.[14, 29, 30]

The effects of stress on less well-vascularised areas is also evident in sportsmen, particularly in the case of hyaline cartilage and intervertebral discs. The gradual diminution of these tissues is accelerated in the case of sportsmen putting heavy loads through the joints concerned – particularly in the case of weightlifters. Correct techniques can minimise, but not negate, these effects.

Nervous adaptation

The reactions of the nervous system of the sportsman to training are best viewed in three categories – integrative, threshold and set point.

Integrative adaptation occurs through a conditioning of reflexes and a patterning of responses. With many repetitions of a stimulus and its response, the integration of the input and output signals is achieved at lower levels of consciousness or at lower levels of subconscious involvement. This repetitive type of training is obvious in the learning of complex skill patterns, but on a physiological level is just as fundamental to the acquisition of greater efficiency within motor functions ranging from postural reflexes to locomotor patterns. For example, a beginner at racewalking will find the normal mode of progression a very difficult and tiring voluntary business. With many hundreds of thousands of repetitions of the racewalking stride it becomes a subconscious and extremely efficient mode of locomotion.

Threshold adaptation occurs in the gradual desensitisation of sensory nerves by exposure to high excitation for great periods of time. The threshold level at which pain occurs, for example, can be trained by exposure – and also by conditioning of the psyche. [22] Many of the effects of strenuous training in (particularly) the anaerobic events are concerned with raising the pain threshold. Pain thresholds also respond to an adaptation in the case of chronic injuries; over a period of time the sportsman unconsciously and also perhaps consciously adapts his receptor mechanisms to be less responsive to the painful stimuli from an injury.

Set point adaptation has been mentioned in the previous chapter. Not only may a sportsman alter his basal set points over a long period of training (e.g. heart rate), but he can also alter the temporary set points which are established at different levels of activity (e.g. core temperature of marathon runners).

Environmental adaptation

Whereas the earlier part of this chapter has been concerned with the sportsman's adaptation to increasing levels of physical work and complexity of task, and his reactions to these, this section is concerned with the physiological adaptation to be gained through training in an environmental stress. Such stresses are generally altitude and temperature.

Altitude

The suddenness with which sports scientists were precipitated into discovering about high altitude in order to enhance athletes' performances at the Mexico Olympics created a situation where wishful rather than constructive thinking seemed to produce results. Some of the major findings have been debunked at the annual meeting of the British Association of Sport and Medicine in 1973. It would be as well for the student to forget previous conceptions, and ignore the fact that a sudden crop of Olympic running champions seemed to have spent their lives on tops of mountains.

At the altitude of Mexico City (2300 m) the barometric pressure is about 80 per cent of the sea-level reading. Athletes unaccustomed to such conditions might expect decrements in performance concomitant with those shown in Table 4.1 (p. 132).[4] The basic hypothesis on the effects of altitude stress as part of the adaptation is that it causes an improvement in the absolute cardiorespiratory function of the sportsman which:

(1) allows him to perform better at altitude than he might otherwise have done; and
(2) gives him an enhancement of his performance upon returning to compete at sea level.

On exposure to lower barometric pressures a sportsman experiences hypoxic hypoxia, i.e. a decrease of the oxygen content in arterial blood (hypoxia) caused by decreased oxygen partial pressure in inspired air (hypoxic). The sensitivity of the carotid and aortic bodies to anoxia stimulates the respiratory centre to increase ventilation, which does not fully restore the oxygen levels but does depress the blood carbon dioxide. The blood pH equilibrates by an increase of kidney bicarbonate extraction and excretion. This excretion of bicarbonate is accompanied by a decrease in plasma volume and, since the total haemoglobin remains unchanged, the *proportion* of haemoglobin will at first increase. This is followed during acclimatisation by a normalising of plasma volume, and an increase in total haemoglobin.[1]

At submaximal work levels the oxygen requirement remains the same for given work loads, and the sportsman compensates by increasing his ventilation rate (see Fig. 4.10, p. 131).[2] After acclimatisation this increase in ventilation rate gradually declines, as does work heart rate, while stroke volume may decrease to a value below that of sea level. Cardiac output at rest and during submaximal work returns

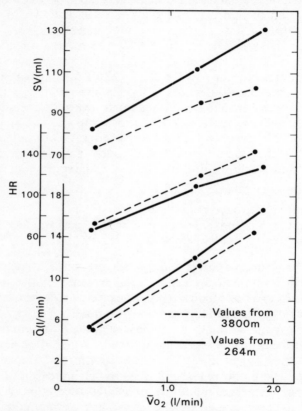

Fig. 7.2 Stroke volume (SV), heart rate (HR) and cardiac output (Q) after 3–4 weeks of acclimatisation to 3800 m, plotted against oxygen consumption (V_{O_2})

Dots represent mean values from 5 subjects in the rest experiments and mean values from 3 subjects at each work level

to almost normal levels after a month's acclimatisation (Fig. 7.2).[18]

During maximal work, top-class athletes when arriving at altitude suffer a decrease in maximal oxygen uptake, which is probably due to a ventilatory limitation since even a 3 l per min oxygen uptake demands a doubling of ventilation rate at 4000 m. Athletes are not as affected as normal subjects, probably because of the greater compliance of their ventilation. There is then a gradual recuperation, which is still not complete after four weeks of acclimatisation. Mountaineers who are exposed to very long periods at high altitude and strenuous work routines (six months or more) experience an increase in total blood volume, and an improvement in the oxygen dissociation mechanisms.[10]

The first point appears to be proven – that athletes exposed to altitude-stress training improve their total circulatory–respiratory system for tissue oxygenation, at both maximal and submaximal work levels, though never reaching their sea-level capacity since their capacity for maintaining sea-level training schedules is diminished. This acclimatisation requires approximately one month of altitude training.

The second point is slightly different, since it is not acclimatisation for acclimatisation's sake, but as a training stressor to improve overall physical capacity. Several nations have established high-altitude training camps for this reason, and the IOC have instituted regulations controlling the attendance periods for sportsmen at such camps. However, there is general agreement among physiologists that athletes in peak training are not likely to improve their sea-level or medium-altitude capacities by training at high altitudes.[3, 7, 13, 27, 32] Altitude training, therefore, is beneficial for acclimatising those who are to compete at altitude, but probably not beneficial for competition at low altitude.

Temperature

In this case, stress adaptation training is almost invariably performed as an acclimatisation process for its own sake.

Little is known about the effects of extreme temperature acclimatisation on sports performance in normal temperatures.

The losses of body heat by the sportsman have been covered in Chapter 6. The heat flow by conduction and radiation into the surrounding air is dependent on the temperature gradient between the skin and the air. The warmer the air, the less does the gradient favour body heat loss. If the surrounding temperature is *higher* than the body temperature, the sportsman will tend to *gain* heat from the environment. Evaporation is then the only means of losing the massive heat production of the body.

The physiological adaptation to heat stress can be seen in two stages. During the first stage there is venous constriction associated with a cutaneous vasodilation. An increased cardiac output is thus shunted to the body periphery, allowing an increased heat loss. There is also an increased sweating rate which assists in dissipating the heat. The first stage lasts for a few days, when it is followed by a disappearance of the venous constriction and capillary blood shunt.[31] The sweat mechanism adjusts to the new set point, greatly increasing its output, and the proportionate salt content in sweat is reduced in order to conserve body electrolyte levels. The athlete should assist his physiological adaptation by ensuring an adequate and constant water replacement − since the body is not widely tolerant of dehydration − and an ingestion of salt, at the times of greatest sweating rather than before or after of these periods.

There are critical time periods of high temperature adaptation.

Period	Adaptation	Methods
1–2 days	none	
2–10 days	up to 90 per cent adapted [26]	short intermittent work periods in the heat up to maximum of 4 hours daily [6, 20]
14 days	loss of adaptation	no exposure to high temperatures
4–7 days	regaining of adaptation [20]	as for adaptation

Sportsmen who are in good condition adapt more quickly than the less fit, but the adaptation procedure ought to proceed by gradual increments of work and heat stress.[32] Overtraining in temperatures hotter than those expected in competition will facilitate performance. The effect of heat on the unadapted competitor is so severe that it is extremely unwise for a sportsman not to prepare himself fully —either by a sufficiently long acclimatising period at the competition site, or by including high temperature training within his own environment.

The initial adaptations to cold are vasoconstriction in the periphery, an increase in basal metabolic rate and generation of body heat by shivering. These effects are almost immediate. In sports performance, individuals will normally solve their body heat conservation problems by wearing appropriate clothing. However, this action is hardly possible in the case of competitive swimming. Other water activities are commonly carried out wearing insulating wet suits, but the only covering commonly worn by swimmers is a smearing of grease or petroleum jelly in long distance swimming, which can be of value in preserving body heat.[24]

One of the major adaptive mechanisms of swimmers, particularly long distance swimmers, is to accumulate adipose fat in order to reduce peripheral circulation and to provide an insulating coat for the body.[9] It has been calculated that each millimetre of subcutaneous fat is equivalent to a temperature rise of $1 \cdot 5$ °C, which is an important mechanism for prevention of hypothermia during swimming,[24] and for increasing the tolerance of low skin temperatures.[23]

Also of importance to swimmers is the habituation response of the sensory threshold to cold. Repeated immersion in very cold water becomes progressively less perceived by the swimmer.

General conclusions

Stress in sport can be experienced in two ways via the sensory nervous system:

(1) subconscious arrival at limiting levels of any performance parameter;

(2) conscious sensations of physical distress arising from
(1).

Adaptive training in sport tackles both of these problems by
seeking a real change in (1) through normal body mechanisms
and by developing new sensory thresholds and tolerance of
distress at exhaustion.

Experiments in adaptation

Most of the *systems* covered in this chapter have already been
described in previous chapters, and suitable experiments will
be possible within the frameworks proposed on those oc-
casions. At this stage, students should be more concerned
with noting *real adaptive* changes, which in general occur
over relatively long periods of time. On a test–retest basis
with the same subjects (which are the most valid experiments)
the time constraints of the experiment may be insufficient to
permit detectable changes. Tests between different subgroups
of subjects can be performed with fewer temporal problems,
but great care is needed in matching subgroups and statis-
tically analysing the data.

The reader is referred to p. 248 for a reminder of suitable
experiment construction, and is advised that parameters may
be divided into certain subgroups. One or more items from
each group *may* be examined on one experiment, with *all*
groups being investigated or one or more groups held constant during the experiment. Where constancy cannot be assured, then assumptions about fluctuations may be made by
referring to standard tests, and their descriptions of such
fluctuations. On a within subjects basis (test–retest) such
assumptions are less critical.

Stressors:

(a) force (magnitude, repetitions, duration, etc.);

(b) temperature (absolute, relative, fluctuations);

(c) humidity;

(d) noise (discrete, random, frequency, volume);

(e) light (spectrum, intensity);

(f) drugs – under medical supervision only;

(g) barometric pressure (altitude, depth, underwater);

(h) sleep deprivation;

(i) wind;

(j) emotion (stimulation, depression, etc.);

(k) diet;

(l) rhythmic fluctuations.

Parameters:

(a) muscle (power and endurance, size, flexibility, tone);

(b) heart (rate, output, size, acceleration, recovery);

(c) lungs (rate, depth, volume, power);

(d) respiration (Vo_2, inspiratory oxygen uptake, carbon dioxide production);

(e) digestion (discomfort, delay, quantity);

(f) sweating (quantity, salt content);

(g) sensory (thresholds, subjective perception);

(h) integration (stimulus – response times, accuracy);

(i) motor (skill, balance).

Stress modes:

(a) continual;

(b) intermittent;

(c) constant magnitude or changing;

(d) duration.

Groups:

(a) sports type;

(b) sex;

(c) age;

(d) anthropometric;

(e) intelligence;

(f) sports ability;

(g) fitness level;

(h) control.

246   Exercise Physiology

References

1. ASMUSSEN, E. and CONSOLAZIO, F. C. (1941) 'The circulation in rest and work on Mount Evans (4300 m)'. *American Journal of Physiology*, **132**, 555.
2. ASTRAND, P. O. (1954) 'The respiratory activity in man exposed to prolonged hypoxia'. *Acta physiologica Scandinavica*, **30**, 343.
3. ASTRAND, P. O. (1966) 'Circulatory and respiratory response to acute and prolonged hypoxia during heavy exercise'. *Schweizerische Zeitschrift fur Sportmedizin*, **14**, 16.
4. BALKE, B. 'Effects of altitude variations on performance'. In, *Exercise Physiology*, Academic Press: New York.
5. BARNARD, R. J. *et al.* (1970) 'Effect of exercise on skeletal muscle'. *Journal of Applied Physiology*, **28**, 762.
6. BEAN, W. B. and EICHNA, L. W. (1943) 'Performance in relation to environmental temperature'. *Federation Proceedings. Federation of American Societies for Experimental Biology*, **2**, 144.
7. BUSKIRK, E. R. *et al.* (1966) 'Physiology and performance of track athletes at various altitudes in the U.S. and Peru'. In, *Proceedings of the International Symposium on Effects of Altitude on Physical Performance*. Alberquerque, New Mexico.
8. CURETON, T. K. (1969) *The physiological effects of exercise programs on adults*. Charles C. Thomas: Springfield, Ill.
9. EDMAN, M. (1964) 'Nutrition and climate'. In, *Medical climatology*. Licht: New Haven, Conn.
10. FERRIS, B. G. (1971) 'Mountaineering'. In, *Encyclopedia of sport science and medicine*. Macmillan: New York.
11. GOLLNICK, P. D. and KING, D. W. (1969) 'Effect of exercise and training on mitochondria of rat skeletal muscle'. *American Journal of Physiology*, **216**, 1502.
12. GOLLNICK, P. D. *et al.* (1971) 'Ultrastructural and enzyme changes in muscles with exercise'. In, *Muscle metabolism during exercise*. Plenum Press: New York.
13. GROVER, R. F. and REEVES, J. T. (1966) 'Exercise performance of athletes at sea level and 3100 m. altitude'. In, *Proceedings of the International Symposium on Effect of Altitude on Physical Performance*. Alberquerque, New Mexico.
14. HEIKKINEN, E. (1972) 'Effects of age and physical training on the development and metabolism of connective tissues'. In, *Proceedings of the Olympic Congress*. Munich.
15. HOLLOSZY, J. O. *et al.* (1970) 'Biochemical adaptations to endurance

exercise in skeletal muscle'. *Proceedings of Symposium on Muscle Metabolism during Exercise*, Karolinska Institute; Stockholm.

16. ISSEKUTZ, B. *et al.* (1965) 'Aerobic work capacity and plasma FFA turnover'. *Journal of Applied Physiology*, **20**, 293.

17. KIESSLING, K. H. *et al.* (1971) 'Effect of physical training on ultrastructural features in human skeletal muscle'. In, *Muscle metabolism during exercise*. Plenum Press: New York.

18. KLAUSEN, K. (1966) 'Cardiac output in man in rest and work during and after acclimatisation to 3,800 m'. *Journal of Applied Physiology*, **21**, 609.

19. KRAUS, H., KIRSTEN, R. and WOLF, J. R. (1969) *Pflugers Archiv für die gesamte Physiologie des Menschen und der Tiere*, **308**, 57.

20. LIND, A. R. and BASS, D. E. (1963) 'The optimal exposure time for the development of acclimatisation to heat'. *Federation Proceedings. Federation of American Societies for Experimental Biology*, **22**, 704.

21. MORGAN, T. E. *et al.* (1971) 'Effects of long term exercise on human muscle mitochondria'. In, *Muscle metabolism during exercise*, Plenum Press: New York.

22. PRESCOTT, F. (1964) *The control of pain*. English Universities Press: London.

23. PUGH, L. G. C. E. and EDHOLM, O. G. (1955) 'The physiology of channel swimmers'. *Lancet*, **269**, 761.

24. PUGH, L. G. C. E. *et al.* (1960) 'A physiological study of channel swimming'. *Clinical Science*, **9**, 257.

25. PUGH, L. G. C. E. (1967) 'Athletes at altitude'. *Journal of Physiology*, **192**, 619.

26. ROBINSON, S. *et al.* (1950) 'Effects of desoxycorticosterone acetate on acclimatisation of men to heat'. *Journal of Applied Physiology*, **2**, 399.

27. SALTIN, B. (1966) 'Aerobic and anaerobic work capacity at an altitude of 2250 m'. In, *Proceedings of the International Symposium on Effects of Altitude on Physical Performance*, Alberquerque, New Mexico.

28. SELYE, H. (1956) *The stress of life*. McGraw-Hill: New York.

29. TIPTON, C. M. *et al.* (1967) 'Influence of physical activity on the strength of knee ligaments in rats'. *American Journal of Physiology*, **212**, 783.

30. VIDIK, A. (1969) *Acta orthopaedica scandinavica*, **40**, 261.

31. WOOD, J. E. and BASS, D. E. (1960) 'Responses of the veins and arterioles of the forearm to walking during acclimatisation to heat in man'. *Journal of Clinical Investigation*, **39**, 825.

32. WYNDHAM, C. H. *et al.* (1960) 'The temperature responses of men after two methods of acclimatisation'. *Arbeitsphysiologie*, **18**, 112.

Experimental work

Students of sports physiology should undertake a great deal of experimental work, in view of the essentially practical nature of their profession. In my opinion, formal lecture time should be backed up by at least double that amount of experimental time. Within this text some suggestions have been made concerning suitable experimental areas. The difficulty of giving specific experiments to be performed is that only a few may be outlined, leaving most unmentioned.

The situations within which experiments may be performed are so specific to each educational environment that, inevitably, set experiments would be greatly adapted or merely ignored. Instead, it has been decided to suggest a basic approach within which a range of experiments may be constructed when the occasion arises.

The experimental approach

An experiment is a situation in which the relation between one or more independent variables, which may or may not have constant values attached to them, and one or more dependent variables with which they are linked, can be investigated. In a situation as complex as physical exercise and the responses to it, there is great difficulty in deciding which are the dependent variables. Generally speaking, variables such as work levels, environmental factors and group characteristics of subjects may be taken as independent since their levels may either be controlled within the experimental situation, or their fluctuations recorded as they occur. The dependent variables are those which change following changes in the independent variables.

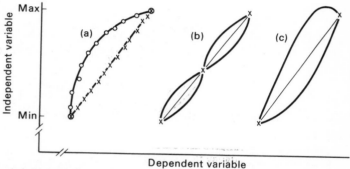

Fig. A.1 Interpolation curves

The relationship between the variables can then be called a physiological rule which applies to the specific conditions under which the experiment is performed. If a sufficient number of conditions is studied, the rule may eventually be generalised across the whole spectrum of conditions. The student ought to be warned that to generalise rules completely is the exception within exercise physiology. To do so involves not only taking a sufficient number of intermediate points, but also examining both extremes of the range. Extremes of sporting performance are very difficult to reach, especially in the non-competitive situation, and when achieved prove to be most trying conditions within which to measure physiological variables. However, if these obstacles are overcome there may be a possibility of generalisation through interpolation (Fig. A.1).

Situation (a) is one in which the experimenter might be

justified in generalising by interpolating between the points to provide more or less regular lines of relationship between the variables; (b) demonstrates the danger of interpolating between two few points, where any one of the three curves might in fact be correct – a situation which is caricatured in (c) where straight line interpolation between two points is quite obviously liable to ridiculous errors.

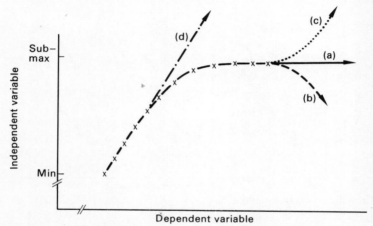

Fig. A.2 Extrapolation curves

Even greater problems arise from extrapolation from data, where, either a line is hypothetically projected beyond its experimental limits or relations established in one field are assumed to be valid outside it – practices unfortunately too common in physiology where animal experiments are extrapolated to the human, and results for ordinary people to the athlete.

The greatest of these extrapolation errors in recent history related to 'maximum' exercise heart rate (see Chapter 3). Fig. A.2 illustrates the problem.

In this case there is a typical straight-line relation at the beginning, which rounds off to a plateau. Extrapolation suggests that for those capable of carrying on beyond the experimental end point, their curves would be of (a) or (b) types.

Unfortunately, the 'superhuman' sportsman has frequently upset the applecart by recording curves like (c), which indicates a marshalling of reserves, and (d) which is a more acceptable continuation of the straight line relationship. One is reminded of the fabled student who drew a graph extrapolated from a single point saying that 'that was the way it ought to go'.

Error

Physiology is rarely an exact science. Most measurements are liable to considerable error. It is not unusual for physiologists quite happily to use experimental techniques having an error range of 20 per cent – and they may be quite justified in so doing. A physiological measuring technique with an error range of 2 per cent is considered very accurate. Error may be minimised by taking care in measuring and averaging a great number of readings. When there are large inherent errors, the magnitudes of any changes in the variables *must* be compared with the experimental error to assess their *significance*. This can only be done by using statistical techniques and the reader should consult a statistics text for a description of simple tests which may accompany the experiments arising from this book.

The experiments

At the end of each chapter, except the first, there is a brief description of some specific points which may affect experiments based on that chapter, a basic categorisation of variables, and a listing of variables within each category. This provides a framework within which experiments, simple or of great complexity, may be performed. Measurements requiring standard physiology laboratory techniques are generally excluded since these techniques are extremely varied and not always available to those for whom this book is written. This is not to say that they should not be used, but that the course tutor is best qualified to decide on their inclusion within the experimental procedure. On the other hand, I believe most firmly that much will be learnt by the student using quite simple techniques, and that in so doing the graduates of the future may retain the habit of scientific inquiry even if their careers carry them into situations where sophisticated experimental facilities are unavailable.

Index